Multiple Myeloma

Edited by Ota Fuchs

Published in London, United Kingdom

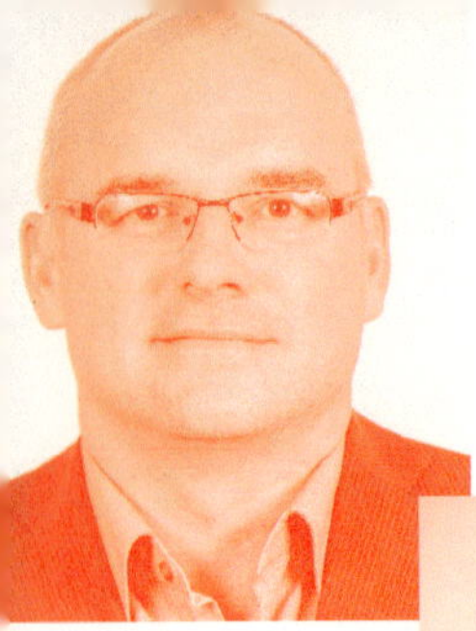
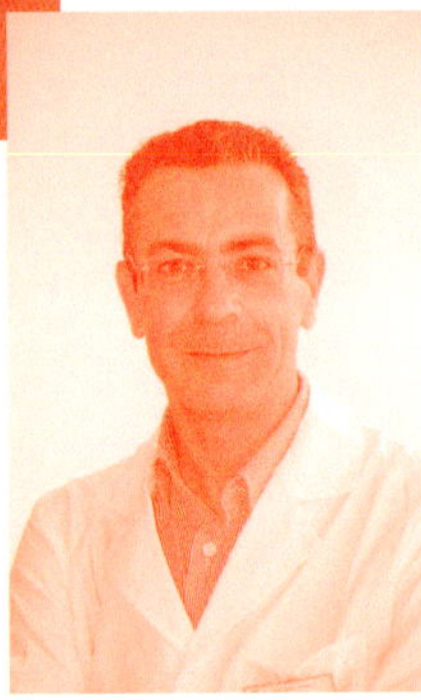
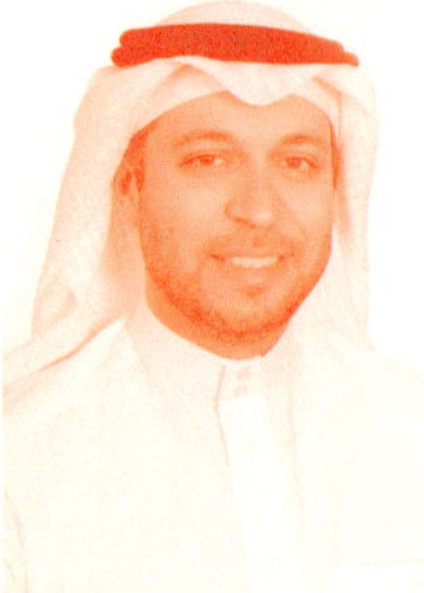
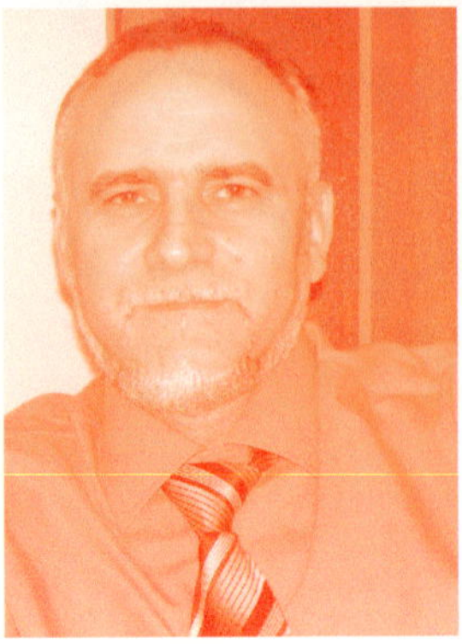
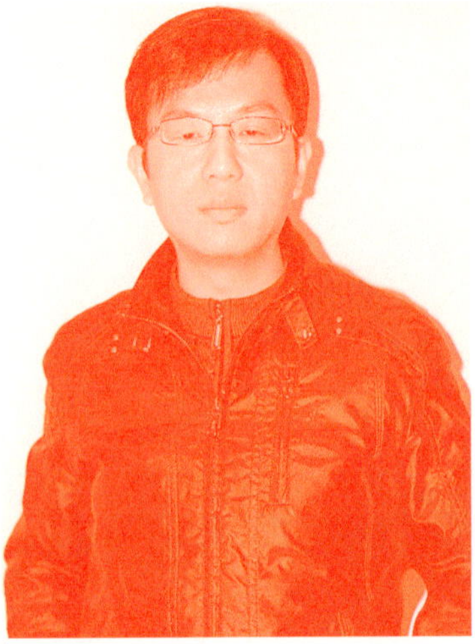
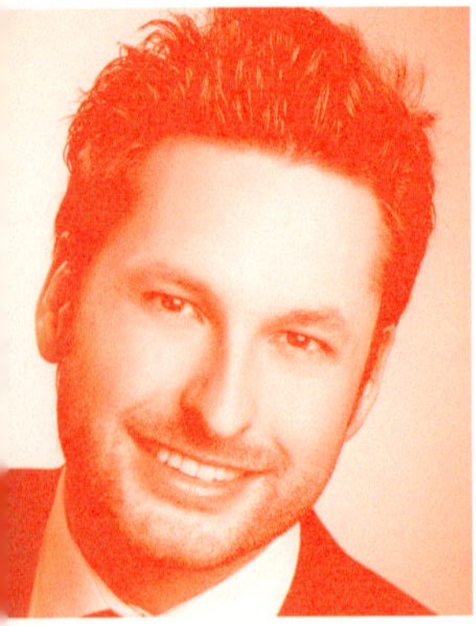
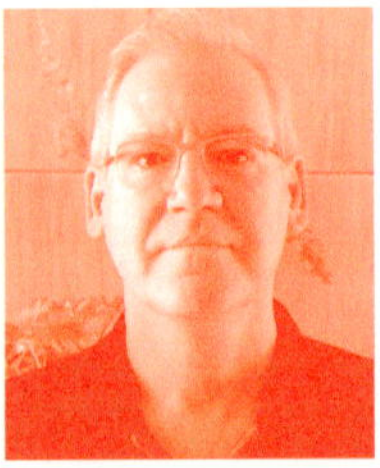

IntechOpen

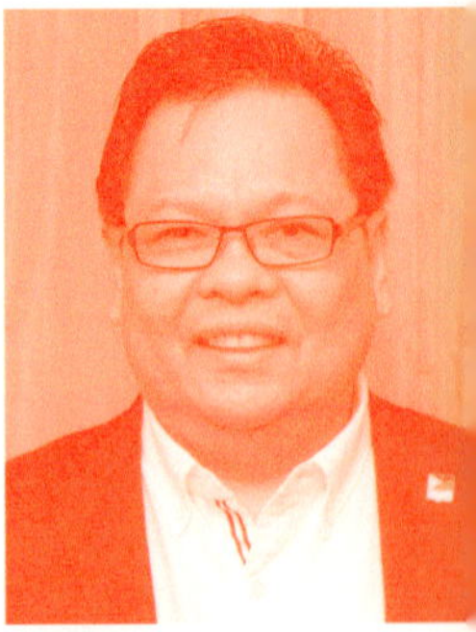
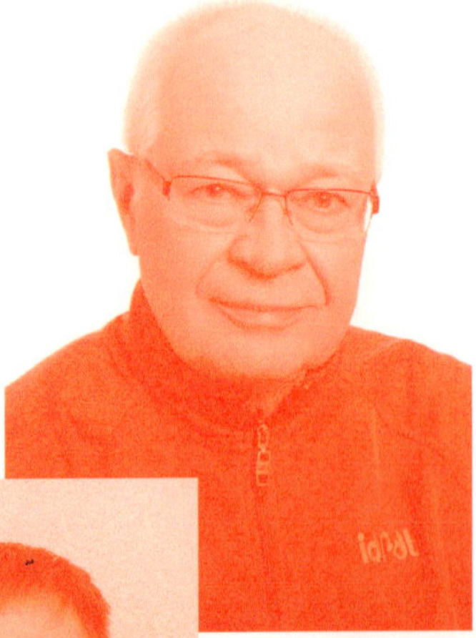
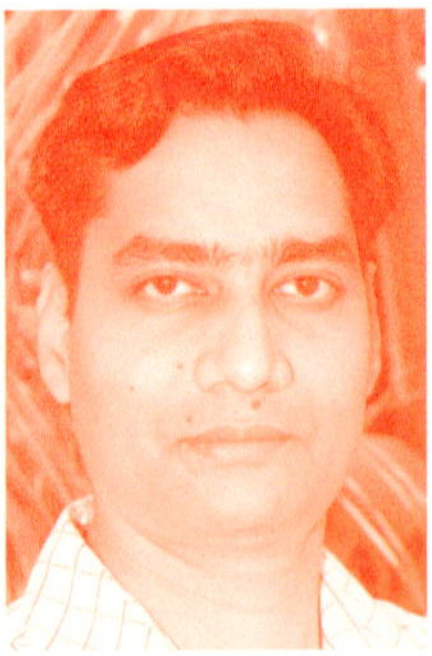
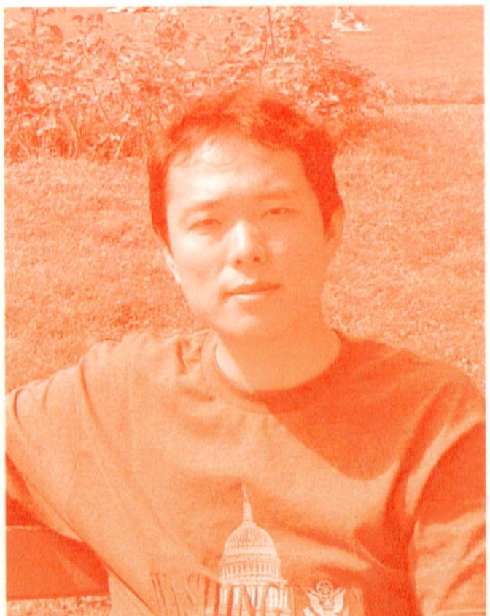
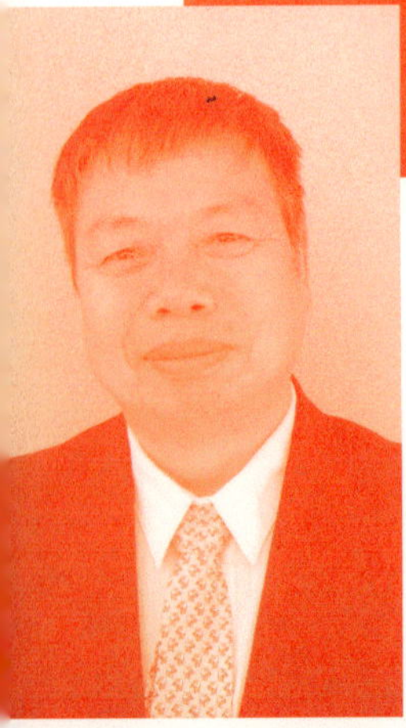
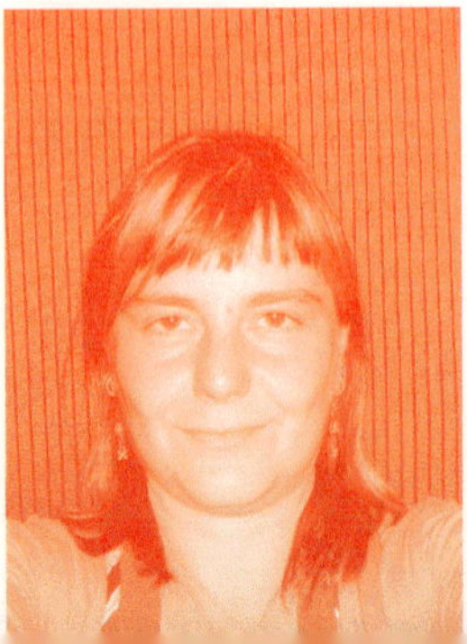

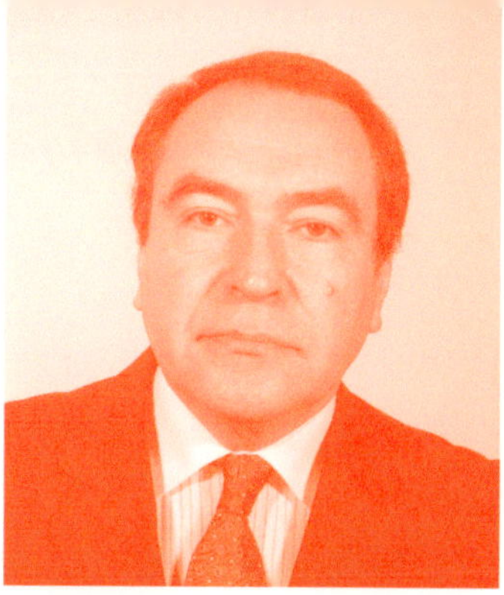
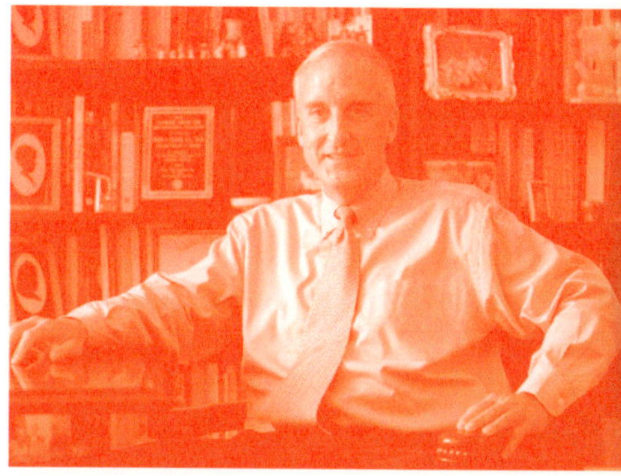
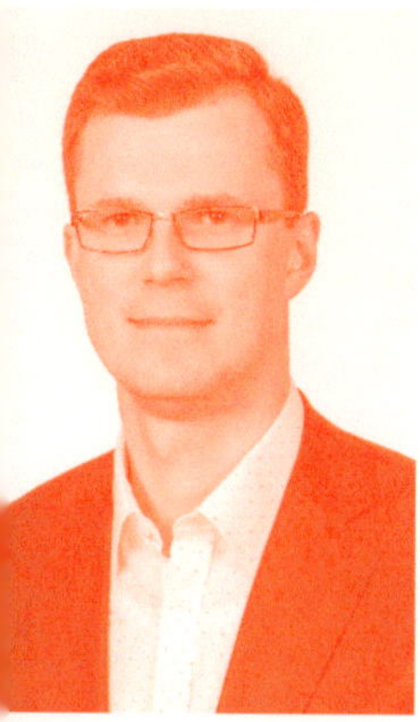
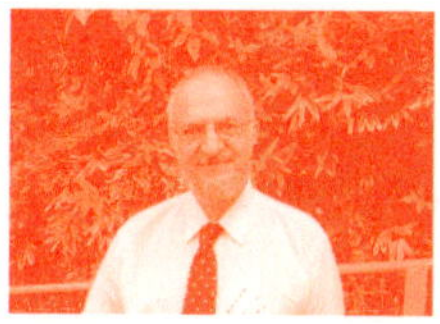
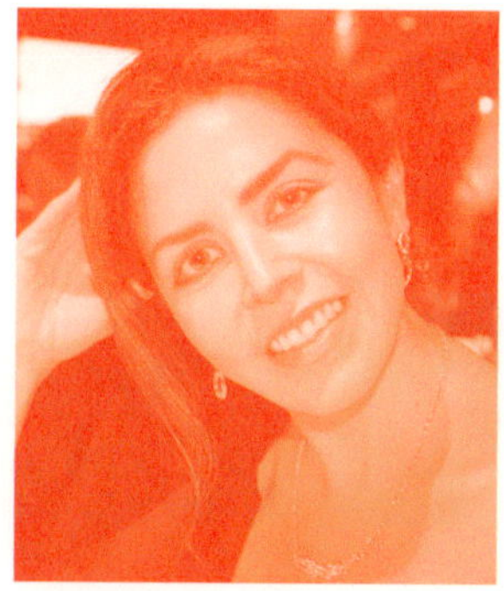

Supporting open minds since 2005

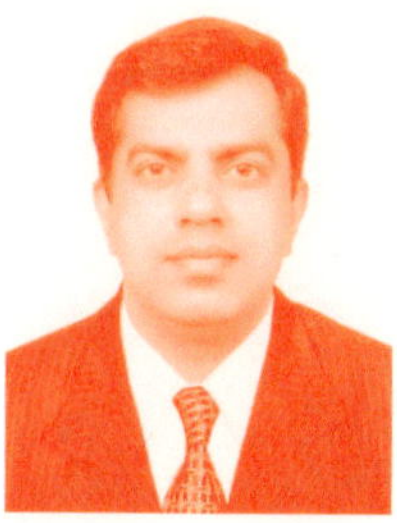
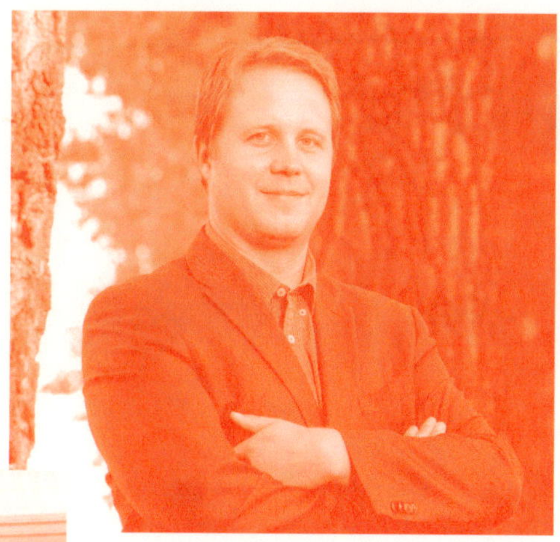
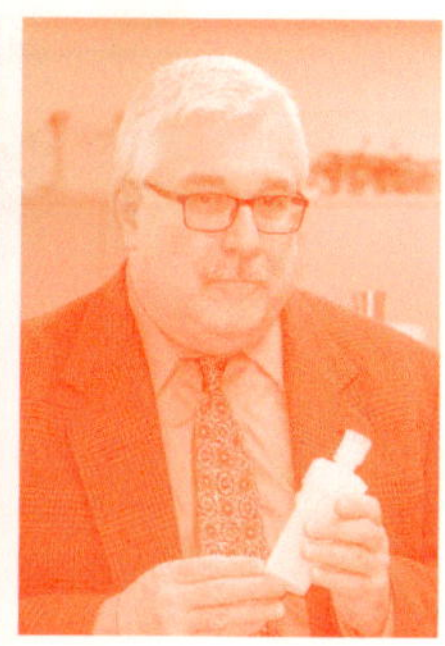
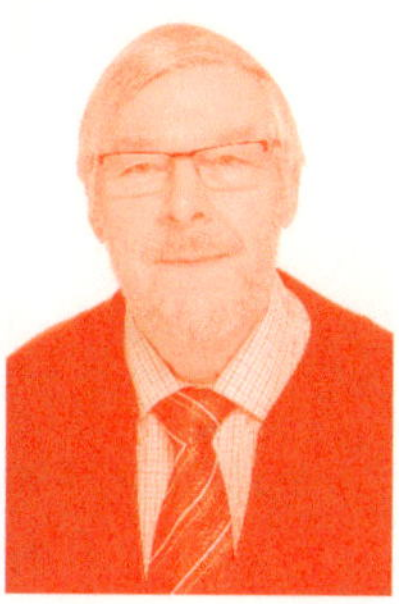
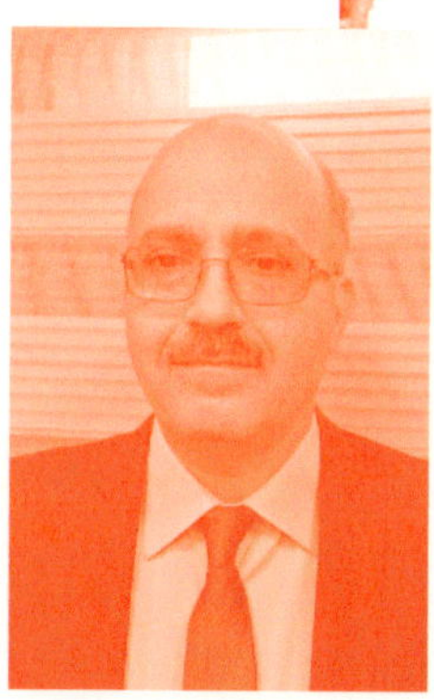
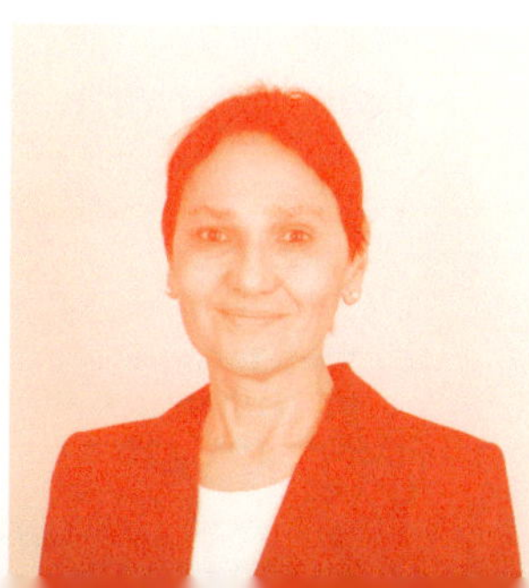
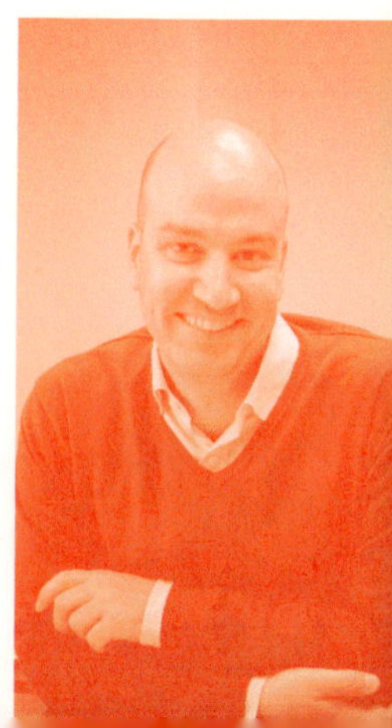

Multiple Myeloma
http://dx.doi.org/10.5772/intechopen.87599
Edited by Ota Fuchs

Contributors
Giulia Palazzo, Howard R. Terebelo, Leo Reap, Maria Teresa Petrucci, Gianfranco Lapietra, Francesca Fazio, Marina Ferrarini, Elisabetta Ferrero, Nikolaos Kanellias, Maria Gavriatopoulou, Evangelos Terpos, Minyahil Alebachew Alebachew Woldu, Atalay Mulu Fentie, Tamrat Assefa Tadesse, Ota Fuchs, Lara Aprile, Giacomo Cecere, Vito Pier Gagliardi, Alessandro Maggi, Antonella Prudenzano, Patrizio Mazza, Magda Marcatti, Fabio Ciceri

First published in London, United Kingdom, 2021 by IntechOpen
IntechOpen is the global imprint of INTECHOPEN LIMITED, registered in England and Wales, registration number: 11086078, 5 Princes Gate Court, London, SW7 2QJ, United Kingdom
Printed in Croatia

British Library Cataloguing-in-Publication Data
A catalogue record for this book is available from the British Library

Additional hard and PDF copies can be obtained from orders@intechopen.com

Multiple Myeloma
Edited by Ota Fuchs
p. cm.
Print ISBN 978-1-83968-620-7
Online ISBN 978-1-83968-621-4
eBook (PDF) ISBN 978-1-83968-622-1

For EU product safety concerns:
IN TECH d.o.o., Prolaz Marije Krucifikse Kozulić 3, 51000 Rijeka, Croatia, info@intechopen.com or visit our website at intechopen.com.

Meet the editor

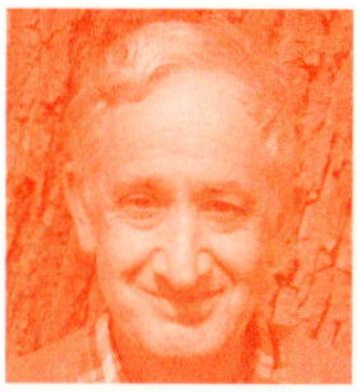

Ota Fuchs graduated from the Chemical Technological University, Prague, Czech Republic, in 1971. He obtained his Ph.D. in Biochemistry from the Faculty of Natural Sciences, Charles University, Prague, in 1981. He is employed as a Senior Scientist at the Institute of Hematology and Blood Transfusion, Prague. He undertook as visiting scientist short-term affiliations at the Beatson Institute for Cancer Research, Glasgow, UK; Institute of Experimental Medicine of the Russian Academy of Medical Sciences in St Peterburg, Russia; and Lady Davis Institute for Medical Research, Jewish General Hospital, Montreal, Canada. Dr. Fuchs was the principal investigator of five projects of the Internal Grant Agency of the Ministry of Health of the Czech Republic and one grant project of the Grant Agency of Czech Republic.

Contents

Preface

Multiple myeloma is a malignant disease characterized by the proliferation of clonal plasma cells in the bone marrow and by the secretion of monoclonal immunoglobulins detected in the serum or urine. Considerable advances have been made in understanding the biology of multiple myeloma through the study of the bone marrow microenvironment. The bone marrow niche appears to play an important role in differentiation, migration, proliferation, survival, and drug resistance of the malignant plasma cells. In multiple myeloma, malignant plasma cells colonize and modify the bone marrow microenvironment through cytokine production and interactions with other cell types. Multiple myeloma cells induce myeloid-derived suppressor cells (MDSC) development and survival. MDSCs promote tumor growth and induce immune suppression. Moreover, antimyeloma therapies such as dexamethasone, melphalan, cyclophosphamide, or immunomodulatory drugs can expand and potentiate MDSC immunosuppressive effects. In contrast to these agents, daratumumab depletes MDSCs. Therefore, MDSC suppression could become an important strategy for potentiation of the efficacy of novel immunotherapies (e.g., chimeric antigen receptor T cells or T-cell engager bispecific antibodies). Daratumumab, a CD38 antagonist, functions through different mechanisms of action including an immune-mediated effect (antibody-dependent cytotoxicity; complement-dependent cytotoxicity; antibody-dependent phagocytosis). It can also cause apoptosis through a direct antitumor effect. New findings have helped the development of novel therapeutic drugs for use in combination with cytostatic therapy. Engineering a proper transgenic mouse model for multiple myeloma is very important for understanding biology by defining the relevance of specific genetic lesions in tumorigenesis and the interaction between malignant cells and their surrounding microenvironment. This book discusses all these areas. The introductory chapter deals with selinexor, approved in combination with dexamethasone at earlier relapse. Chapter 2 provides a review of prognostic and predictive factors in newly diagnosed multiple myeloma. Chapter 3 discusses treatment approaches for multiple myeloma. Chapters 4–6 introduce antibody therapies for multiple myeloma and, finally, Chapter 7 analyzes three-dimensional (3D) models mimicking multiple myeloma bone marrow–microenvironment interactions.

Ota Fuchs, PhD
Institute of Hematology and Blood Transfusion,
Department of Genomics,
Prague, Czech Republic

Chapter 1

Introductory Chapter: Oral Selinexor, a Selective Inhibitor of Nuclear Export in the Treatment of Patients with Multiple Myeloma Refractory to Proteasome Inhibitors, Immunomodulatory Agents and Monoclonal Antibodies

Ota Fuchs

1. Introduction

The export of proteins from the nucleus to the cytoplasm plays an important role in the development of cancer and drug resistance [1–3]. The major mammalian nuclear export receptor protein is exportin 1 (XPO1, also known as chromosomal maintenance 1/ CRM1/) [1–5]. The crystal structure of this protein showed a complex with the Ran protein (Ras-related nuclear protein) bound to GTP [6, 7]. XPO1 interacts also with nucleoporins in the nuclear pore complex and transports multiple tumor suppressor proteins (eg p53, FOXO, p21 pRB, BRCA1/2), growth regulators, and oncoprotein mRNAs (eg c-myc, Bcl-xL, MDM2, cyclins) containing a leucine rich nuclear export signal (NES) (**Figure 1**) [8]. XPO1 is also involved in regulation of cytoplasmic localization and translation of c-myc and other oncoprotein mRNAs (eg cyclin D1, Bcl-6, Mdm2, and Pim) through complexing with eukaryotic initiation factor 4E (eIF4E) [9]. The XPO1 protein level is increased in many types of cancer including multiple myeloma [10–13]. As a result of the increased nuclear-cytoplasmic transport in cancer cells, an elevated level of multiple tumor suppressor proteins and oncoproteins in the cytoplasm leads to advanced disease, resistance to therapy, and poor survival. Thus, XPO1 is a promising cancer drug target. Leptomycin B (LMB) is a Streptomyces metabolite that inhibits the function of XPO1 in NES-dependent nuclear export of proteins [14]. However, clinical studies found serious side effects of LMB. In order to find a more specific inhibitor of XPO1 without side effects, many natural and synthetic compounds have been tested. These compounds include selinexor (KPT-330, XPOVIO™), verdinexor (KPT-335), KPT-185, KPT-276, KPT-251, and KPT-8602 [15–18]. These agents are a family of small molecules that block nuclear export through covalent

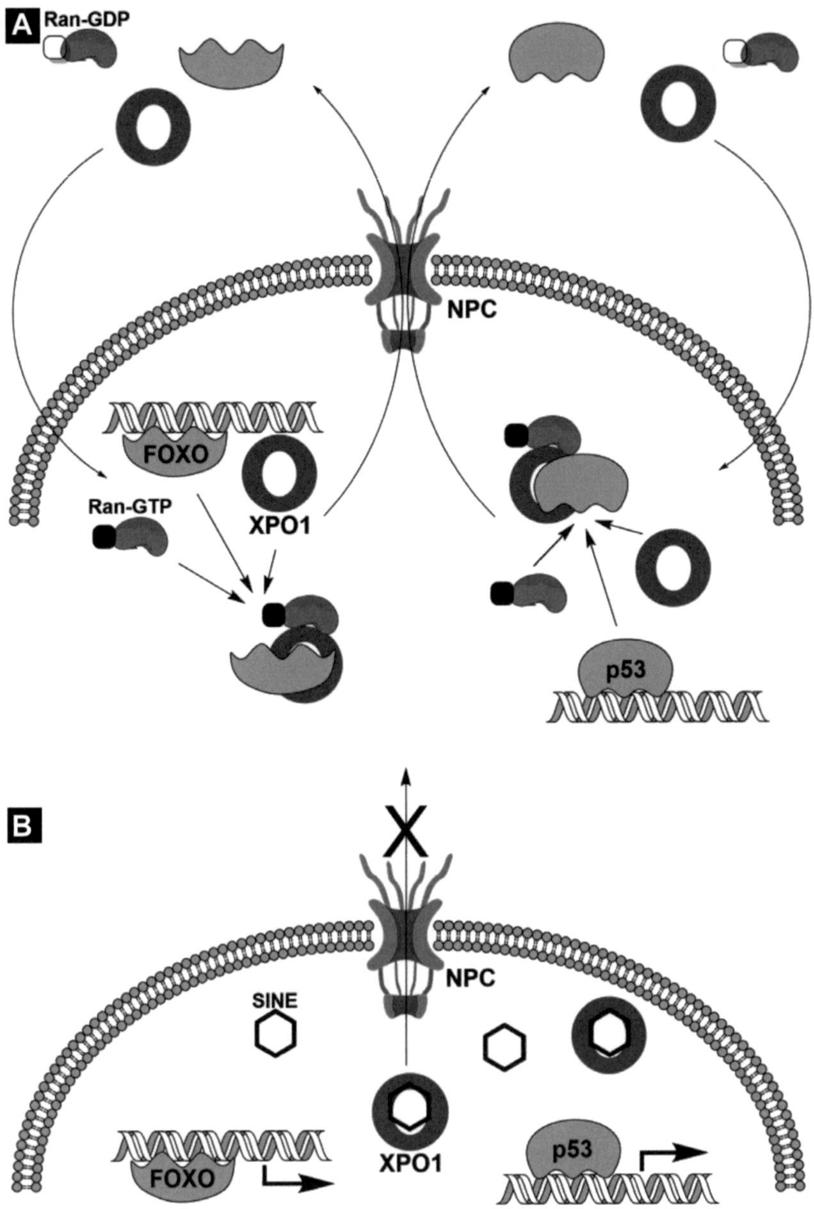

Figure 1.
Exportin 1-mediated nuclear export in multiple myeloma; Abbreviations: Ran-GDP and Ran-GTP – GDP or GTP bound Ras related factor; NPC – nuclear pore complex; SINE - selective inhibitor of nuclear export; FOXO – a subgroup of the Forkhead family of transcription factors, p53 – a tumor suppressor protein and transcription factor; XPO1 – exportin 1, also known as chromosomal maintenance 1 (CRM1); (A) XPO1 transports nuclear proteins out of the nucleus. Cargo proteins such as FOXO or p53 that are marked for export from the nucleus bind a pocket in XPO1 in the presence of the activated small G-protein, Ran. The active Ran-GTP-XPO1-cargo complex is exported from the nucleus through the nuclear pore complex driven by the concentration gradient of Ran-GTP across the nuclear membrane. Once in the cytoplasm, Ran-GTP is hydrolyzed to Ran-GDP, and the XPO1-cargo complex dissociates. (B) SINE compounds (Hexagons) bind to XPO1-Cys^{528} *and occupy the cargo-binding pocket of XPO1 and prevent formation of the Ran-GTP-XPO1-cargo complex. The result is increased nuclear localization of tumor suppressor cargo proteins and upregulation of their transcriptional activity [15].*

binding to cysteine 528 (Cys528) in the cargo proteins NES-binding pocket of exportin1 and contribute to cancer cell death [15]. All these drugs have been developed by Karyopharm Therapeutics Inc., Natick, MA.

2. Selinexor-a small molecule exportin 1 inhibitor

The structural formula of selinexor is shown in **Figure 2**. Selinexor is a first member of small molecule oral inhibitors of exportin 1 developed for the treatment of cancer. Selinexor in combination with a synthetic glucocorticoid dexamethasone was approved by the FDA (U.S. Food and Drug Administration) on July 3, 2019 for the treatment of adult patients with relapsed or refractory multiple myeloma (RRMM) who have received at least four prior therapies. Selinexor synergizes with dexamethasone and inhibits the mTOR pathway and subsequently induces cell death in multiple myeloma cells [19]. Selinexor increases the expression of glucocorticoid receptor and in combination with dexamethasone stimulates transcriptional activity of the glucocoticoid receptor [19]. Selinexor is studied in clinical trials also in many hematological and solid cancers [20–24]. The treatment with selinexor in preclinical and clinical studies resulted in nuclear localization of tumor suppressor proteins (eg p53 and FOXO3A), induced apoptosis and decreased proliferation. Selinexor reduces the expression of DNA damage repair proteins and sensitizes cancer cells to DNA damaging agents [25]. Selinexor blocks the transcription factor NF-κB and induces ribosomal stressby disruption of ribosomal subunits assembly [26].

Selinexor is orally bioavailable with a mean half-life 6–8 h after a single dose. Selinexor pharmacokinetics are not significantly affected by age, sex, ethnicity, renal impairment or mild hepatic impairment. Most frequent adverse events associated with selinexor treatment are thrombocytopenia, fatigue, nausea, anemia, decreased appetite, decreased weight, diarrhoea, vomiting, hyponatremia, neutropenia, leukopenia, constipation, dyspnoea, and upper respiratory tract infection.

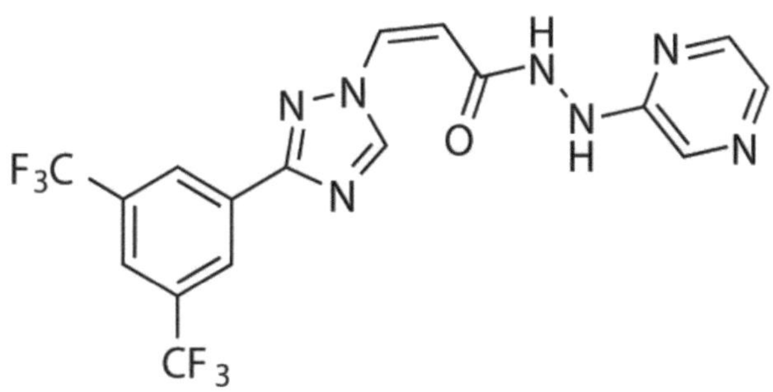

Figure 2.
Chemical structure of selinexor (alternative names: ATG-010, KPT-330, ONO7705, XPOVIO, CRM1 nuclear export inhibitor). Chemical name: (Z)-3-(3-(3,5-bis(trifluoromethyl)phenyl-1H-1,2,4-triazol-1-yl)-N′-(pyrazin-2-yl)acrylohydrazide.

3. The phase II STORM trial with selinexor plus low-dose dexamethasone in patients with multiple myeloma pretreated with bortezomib, carfilzomib, lenalidomide, pomalidomide, daratumumab, and an alkylating agent

Selinexor demonstrated small single-agent activity with an overall response rate achieved in 4% (2/57 heavily pre-treated patients with RRMM (about six prior therapies)) [27]. The response was considerably increased from 4 to 50% (6/12) when selinexor was combined with dexamethasone in a phase I trial in patients with advanced hematological malignancies (NCT 01607892) [27]. The phase II STORM trial (NCT02336815) with selinexor and dexamethasone combination in heavily pre-treated patients with RRMM had relatively quick responses. The primary endpoint was overall response. Patients were given twice weekly oral doses of selinexor (80 mg) and dexamethasone (20 mg) in 28-day cycles [28, 29]. An overall response was recorded in 21% patients (16/78) or 26% (32/122) and median duration of response was 5 months. Patients required a lot of supportive care to mange many side effects. The most common adverse event was thrombocytopenia.

4. A multicenter, open-label, phase 1b/2, dose escalation trial STOMP in patients with relapsed or refractory multiple myeloma with a median of three prior therapies

The STOMP trial (NCT02343042) is a five arms study of selinexor, dexamethasone and either lenalidomide, pomalidomide, bortezomib, carfilzomib or daratumumab for the treatment of relapsed or refractory multiple myeloma with median of three prior therapies in order to evaluate the safety, tolerability and efficacy of these combinations, determining the maximum tolerated dose, the recommended phase 2 dose, overall response rate (ORR), and progression-free survival (PFS) [23, 24, 26]. Individual arms were described in abstracts No. 726, 1366, and 1393 on ASH 2020 meeting.

5. The randomized open-label, phase III international BOSTON trial in patients with relapsed or refractory multiple myeloma with a median of two prior therapies

The combination of selinexor and bortezomib once per week plus dexamethasone twice per week (SVd) was compared with bortezomib twice per week in combination with dexamethasone four times per week for the first six months and one half of this dose thereafter (Vd) [30]. Median PFS was longer with selinexor treatment: 13.93 months versus 9.46 months in the Vd group. The improvements in survival and response rates with selinexor were associated with higher rates of adverse events [30].

This work was supported by the project for conceptual development of research organisation No 00023736 (Institute of Hematology and Blood Transfusion) from the Ministry of Health of the Czech Republic.

Author details

Ota Fuchs
Institute of Hematology and Blood Transfusion, Prague, Czech Republic

*Address all correspondence to: ota.fuchs@uhkt.cz

References

[1] Turner JG, Sullivan DM. CRM1 mediated nuclear export of proteins and drug resistance in cancer. Current Medicinal Chemistry. 2008; **15**(26): 2648-2655. DOI: 10.2174/092986708786242859

[2] Nguen KT, Holloway MP, Altura RA. The CRM1 nuclear export protein in normal development and disease. International Journal of Biochemistry and Molecular Biology. 2012; **3**(2): 137-151. PMID: 22773955/ISSN: 2152-4114/ IJBM 1204001

[3] Turner JG, Dawson J, Cubitt CL, Baz R, Sullivan DM. Inhibition of CRM1-dependent nuclear export sensitizes malignant cells to cytotoxic and targeted agents. Seminars in Cance Biology. 2014; **27**: 62-73. DOI: 10.1016/j. semcancer.2014.03.001

[4] Gravina GL, Senapedis W, Mc Cauley D, Baloglu E, Shacham S, FestucciaC.Nucleo-cytoplasmictransport as a therapeutic target of cancer. Journal of Hematology & Oncology. 2014; **7**: 85. DOI: 10.1186/s13045-014-0085-1

[5] Lu C, Figueroa JA, Liu Z, Konala V, Aulakh A, Verma R, et al. Nuclear export as a novel therapeutic target: the CRM1 connection. Current Cancer Drug Targets. 2015; **15**(7): 575-592. DOI: 10.2174/156800961507150828223554

[6] Monecke T, Güttler T, Neumann P, Dickmanns A, Görlich D, Ficner R. Crystal structure of the nuclear export receptor CRM1 in complex with Snurportin1 and RanGTP. Science. 2009; **324**(5930): 1087-1091. DOI: 10.1126/science.1173388

[7] Monecke T, Dickmanns A, Ficner R. Allosteric control of the exportin CRM1 unraveled by crystal structure analysis. FEBS Journal. 2014; **281**(18): 4179-4194. DOI: 10.1111/febs.12842

[8] Fung HY, Chook YM. Atomic basis of CRM1-cargo recognition, release and inhibition. Seminars in Cancer Biology. 2014; **27**: 52-61. DOI: 10.1016/ semcancer.2014.03.002

[9] Volpon L, Culjkovic-Kraljacic B, Sohn HS, Blanchet-Cohen A, Osborne MJ, Borden KLB. A biochemical framework for eIF4E-dependent mRNA export and nuclear recycling of the export machinery. RNA. 2017; **23**(6): 927-937. DOI: 10.1261/ rna.060137.116

[10] Schmidt J, Braggio E, Kortuem KM, Egan JB, Zhu YX, Xin CS, et al. Genome-wide studies in multiple myeloma identify XPO1/CRM1 as a critical target validated using the selective nuclear export inhibitor KPT-276. Leukemia. 2013; **27**(12): 2357-2365. DOI: 10.1038/leu.2013.172

[11] Muqbil I, Azmi AS, Mohammad RM. Nuclear export inhibition for pancreatic cancer therapy. Cancers (Basel). 2018; **10**(5): 138. DOI: 103390/cancers10050138

[12] Chanukuppa V, Paul D, Taunk K, Chatterjee T, Sharma S, Kumar S, et al. XPO1 is a critical player for bortezomib resistance in multiple myeloma: A quantitative proteomic approach. Journal of Proteomics. 2019; **209**: 103504. DOI: 10.1016/j. prot.2019.103504

[13] Taylor J, Sendino M, Gorelick AN, Pastore A, Chang MT, Penson AV, et al. Altered nuclear export signal recognition as a driver of oncogenesis. Cancer Discovery. 2019; **9**(10): 1452-1467. DOI: 10.1158/2159-8290. CD-19-0298

[14] Kudo N, Wolff B, Sekimoto T, Schreiner EP, Yoneda Y, Yanagida M, et al. Leptomycin B inhibition of signal-mediated nuclear export by direct

binding to CRM1. Experimental Cell Research. 1998; **242**(2): 540-547. DOI: 10.1006/excr.1998.4136

[15] Parikh K, Cang S, Sekhri A, Liu D. Selective inhibitors of nuclear export (SINE)-a novel class of anti-cancer agents. Journal of Hematology & Oncology. 2014; **7**: 78. DOI: 10.1186/s13045-014-0078-0

[16] Gandhi UH, Senapedis W, Baloglu E, Unger TJ, Chari A, Vogl D, Cornell RF. Clinical implications of targeting XPO1-mediated nuclear export in multiple myeloma. Clinical Lymphoma, Myeloma & Leukemia. 2018; **18**(5): 335-345. DOI: 10.1016/j.clml.2018.03.003

[17] Allegra A, Innao V, Allegra AG, Leanza R, Musolino C. Selective inhibitors of nuclear export in the treatment of hematologic malignancies. Clinical Lymphoma, Myeloma & Leukemia. 2019; **19**(11): 689-698. DOI: 10.1016/j.clml.2019.08.011

[18] Nachmias B, Schimmer AD. Targeting nuclear import and export in hematological malignancies. Leukemia. 2020; **34**(11): 2875-2886. DOI: 10.1038/s41375-020-0958-y

[19] Argueta C, Kashyap T, Klebanov B, Unger TJ, Guo C, Harrington S, et al. Selinexor synergizes with dexamethasone to repress mTORC1 signaling and induce multiple myeloma cell death. Oncotarget. 2018; **9**(39): 25529-25544. DOI: 10.18632/oncotarget.25368

[20] Syed YY. Selinexor: first global approval. Drugs. 2019; **79**(13): 1485-1494. DOI: 10.1007/s40265-019-01188-9

[21] Peterson TJ, Orozco J, Buege M. Selinexor: A first-in-class nuclear export inhibitor for management of multiply relapsed multiple myeloma. Annals of Pharmacotherapy. 2020; **54**(6): 577-582. DOI: 10.1177/1060028019892643

[22] Podar K, Shah J, Chari A, Richardson PG, Jagannath S. Selinexor for the treatment of multiple myeloma. Expert Oinion on Pharmacotherapy. 2020; **21**(4): 398-408. DOI: 10.1080/14656566.2019.1707184

[23] Richter J, Madduri D, Richard S, Chari A. Selinexor in relapsed/refractory multiple myeloma. Therapeutic Advances in Hematology. 2020; **11**: 1-10. DOI: 10.1177/2040620720930629

[24] Benkova K, Mihalyova J, Hajek R, Jelinek T. Selinexor, selective inhibitor of nuclear export: unselective bullet for blood cancers. Blood Reviews. 2020; on line ahead of print Sep 15; 100758. DOI: 10.1016/j.blre.2020.100758

[25] Kashyap T, Argueta C, Unger TJ, Klebanov B, Debler S, Senapedis W, et al. Selinexor reduces the expression of DNA damage repair proteins and sensitizes cancer cells to DNA damaging agents. Oncotarget. 2018; **9**(56): 30773-30786. DOI: 10.18632/oncotarget.25637

[26] Bahlis NJ, Sutherland H, White D, Sebag M, Lentzsch S, Kotb R, et al. Selinexor plus low-dose bortezomib and dexamethasone for patients with relapsed or refractory multiple myeloma. Blood. 2018; **132**(24): 2546-2554. DOI: 10.1182/blood-2018-06-858852

[27] Chen C, Siegel D, Guttierrez M, Jacoby M, Hofmeister CC, Gabrail N, et al. Safety and efficacy of selinexor in relapsed or refractory multiple myeloma and Waldenstrom macroglobulinemia. Blood. 2018; **131**(8): 855-863. DOI: 10.1182/blood-2017-08-797886

[28] Vogl DT, Dingli D, Cornell RF, Huff CA, Jagannath S, Bhutani D, et al. Selective inhibition of nuclear export with oral selinexor for treatment of relapsed or refractory multiple myeloma. Journal of Clinical Oncology. 2018; **36**(9): 859-866. DOI: 10.1200/JCO.2017.75.5207

[29] Chari A, Vogl DT, Gavriatopoulou M, Naoka AK, Yee AJ, Huff CA, et al. Oral selinexor-dexamethasone for triple class refractory multiple myeloma. The New England Journal of Medicine 2019; **381**(8): 727-738. DOI: 10.1056/NEJMoa1903455

[30] Grosicki S, Simonova M, Spicka I, Pour L, Kriachok I, Gavriatopoulou M, et al. Once-per-week selinexor, bortezomib, and dexamethasone versus twice-per-week bortezomib dexamethasone in patients with multiple myeloma (BOSTON): a randomised, open-label, phase 3 trial. Lancet. 2020; **396**(10262): 1563-1573. DOI: 10.1016/S0140-6736(20)32292-3.

Chapter 2

Prognostic and Predictive Factors in Newly Diagnosed Multiple Myeloma Patients with Early Mortality with Prediction Matrix and Three and Five-Year Overall Survival

Howard R. Terebelo and Leo Reap

Abstract

Survival rates for newly diagnosed multiple myeloma have increased to a remarkable 8–12 years. Novel agents, autologous stem cell transplantation, monoclonal antibodies, improvements in supportive care and attention to minimal residual disease negative all have aided this remarkable journey. With these treatments we are identifying tools to achieve complete remissions. Prognostic factors have an important role in selecting proper patient approaches for trial designs. Prognostic and predictive clinical biomarkers have shaped staging and treatment selections for newly diagnosed multiple myeloma. Here we review the Early Mortality Prediction Matrix to identify those at risk of an early death (<6 months) incorporating both disease biology with patient fitness. We also review current standards of care for multiple myeloma and provide a three and five-year overall survival prediction matrix. We review benefits for MRD negativity and Next-Gen Sequencing. These tools will help clinicians improve upon reducing early mortality in newly diagnosed multiple myeloma patients and provide further framework for improving survival by assessing clinical, biologic and individual multiple myeloma patients.

Keywords: newly diagnosed multiple myeloma, prediction matrix, prognostic factors, prediction factors, progression-free survival, early mortality, novel agents, next-gen sequencing, overall survival

1. Introduction-early mortality

The current era of advances in multiple myeloma (MM) identifies a subset of newly diagnosed multiple myeloma (NDMM) patients with early mortality (EM) within the first 6 months of diagnosis [1–6].

Prognostic and predictive risk factors have been identified by the International Myeloma Working Group (IMWG) based upon the LDH, international staging system (ISS), Stage III disease and adverse cytogenetics [7]. Limitations of this study include patients limited to autologous stem cell transplantation (SCT) which included only 40% of all patients. Prediction matrix models based upon those created for cardiovascular disease and rheumatoid arthritis [8, 9] which can calculate the risk of specific outcomes such as mortality allowing the differential weighting of risk factors. We can identify patients at risk with NDMM for EM to provide insight in applying different treatment approaches. Prediction tools have been applied in other hematologic malignancies to predict EM. In AML, prediction factors have improved treatment paradigms [10]. In diffuse large B-cell lymphoma, cell of origin and molecular markers along with PET scans have provided earlier treatment interventions to improve outcomes [11, 12].

Real World patients often differ from those enrolled in clinical trials. These patients tend to be older and less fit, have more co-morbidities and less often SCT candidates [13]. An observational patient registry allows broad patient characteristics and treatment outcomes while assessing NDMM patient characteristics, biology, co-morbidities and treatments for progression-free survival (PFS) and overall survival (OS) [13–16].

2. Early mortality in the Connect MM Registry

The Connect MM Registry reported on more than 3000 NDMM to identify and characterize EM. The first cohort included the first 1500 patients. Data was collected from an unselected patient population from routine clinical practices (81% community and 18% academic). Here a prognostic tool to assess the risk of EM based upon weighting of risk factors in elderly, SCT and non-SCT eligible patients was created to construct an Early Mortality Prediction Matrix (EMPM). See **Figure 1.**

For the 102 NDMM patients with EM, 39.2% (2.7% of total enrolled) were due to MM progression and 32.9% were related to non-causes. Common causes of death included heart failure, pneumonia, infections, and renal failure. The other

A

Mobility	PC	ISS	Creat	ECOG ≥ 2, Hypertension = Yes, Age > 75	ECOG ≥ 2, Hypertension = Yes, Age ≤ 75	ECOG ≥ 2, Hypertension = No, Age > 75	ECOG ≥ 2, Hypertension = No, Age ≤ 75	ECOG < 2, Hypertension = Yes, Age > 75	ECOG < 2, Hypertension = Yes, Age ≤ 75	ECOG < 2, Hypertension = No, Age > 75	ECOG < 2, Hypertension = No, Age ≤ 75
Mobility: No problem in walking about	PC > 150	ISS I, II	Creat ≤ 2	12%	8%	7%	4%	3%	2%	2%	1%
			Creat > 2	18%	11%	10%	6%	5%	3%	3%	2%
		ISS III	Creat ≤ 2	20%	13%	12%	7%	6%	4%	3%	2%
			Creat > 2	29%	19%	17%	11%	10%	6%	5%	3%
	PC ≤ 150	ISS I, II	Creat ≤ 2	24%	16%	14%	9%	8%	5%	4%	2%
			Creat > 2	34%	23%	21%	13%	12%	7%	6%	4%
		ISS III	Creat ≤ 2	37%	26%	23%	15%	13%	8%	7%	4%
			Creat > 2	48%	36%	32%	22%	19%	12%	11%	7%
Mobility: some problem in walking about	PC > 150	ISS I, II	Creat ≤ 2	25%	16%	15%	9%	8%	5%	4%	3%
			Creat > 2	35%	24%	21%	14%	12%	7%	7%	4%
		ISS III	Creat ≤ 2	38%	27%	24%	16%	14%	9%	8%	5%
			Creat > 2	50%	37%	34%	23%	20%	13%	11%	7%
	PC ≤ 150	ISS I, II	Creat ≤ 2	43%	31%	28%	19%	16%	10%	9%	6%
			Creat > 2	55%	42%	38%	27%	24%	16%	14%	9%
		ISS III	Creat ≤ 2	59%	46%	42%	30%	27%	18%	16%	10%
			Creat > 2	69%	57%	54%	40%	37%	26%	23%	15%
Mobility: confined to bed	PC > 150	ISS I, II	Creat ≤ 2	45%	32%	29%	19%	17%	11%	10%	6%
			Creat > 2	56%	43%	40%	28%	25%	16%	14%	9%
		ISS III	Creat ≤ 2	60%	47%	43%	31%	28%	18%	16%	10%
			Creat > 2	71%	58%	55%	42%	38%	27%	24%	16%
	PC ≤ 150	ISS I, II	Creat ≤ 2	65%	52%	49%	36%	32%	22%	20%	12%
			Creat > 2	75%	63%	60%	47%	43%	31%	28%	19%
		ISS III	Creat ≤ 2	77%	67%	64%	51%	47%	34%	31%	21%
			Creat > 2	85%	76%	74%	62%	59%	45%	42%	30%

Figure 1.
A color-coded guide for the clinician identifies which patient (in red) who are at highest risk for EM within six months of diagnosis compared to green and yellow patients who are lowest risk.

28.4% died of other causes or unknown. For those patients surviving more than six months causes of deaths were due to MM (58%) with 5% due to non-myeloma causes. The patients with EM received less triplet therapy (30% vs. 44.7%) and more radiation (24.5% vs. 15.3%) compared with longer surviving patients. EM patients were sicker and less likely to receive triplet therapy.

3. Conclusions

Prior to the era of novel agents, the incidence of EM in NDMM was 10–14% [1, 5, 17, 18]. Novel agents, supportive care, and SCT have improved PFS and OS. The promise of CAR-T therapy, monoclonal antibodies and unique agent BCMA directed against tumor necrosis super family member 17 suggest ongoing improvement for NDMM patients. Key management issues and controversies in EM patients in NDMM patients were passionately presented by Gonsalves [19]. Here the authors defined EM occurring in phase III trials and outlined key management issue strategies for NDMM to mitigate EM and summarizing those patients most at risk. The EMPM here describes parameters to identify NDMM patients at risk for EM, pitfalls in treatment and opportunities to formally address EM in clinical trials.

The prognosis of NDMM patients depends upon staging, patient features, disease biology and treatment outcomes [3]. Risk stratification utilizes the Revised-International Staging System (R-ISS) as devised by the IMWG. The R-ISS is applicable for long-term prognosis but cannot identify those at risk for EM with NDMM [20]. Issues with the R-ISS include a point-based system which is disease specific factors which cannot assess the relative individual of each factor and does not account for patient-specific risk factors. The frailty score, as in the R-ISS, is a point-based system that combines age, functional status and co-morbiditites to predict long-term survival and treatment feasibility in elderly patients with NDMM [20]. Combining the frailty score with the R-ISS stage improves the prognostic value for each score to predict long-term survival. However, neither score alone or when combined has been used to predict NDMM patients at highest risk for EM.

Prognostic studies provide clinicians with a better understanding of the relationship in NDMM patients between the aggressiveness of disease and survival. There are significant gaps in our understanding the optimum ways to risk-stratify NDMM patients when incorporating patient and disease-specific risk factors along with combining the relative contributions of individual risk factors. Existing point-based systems make it difficult to accurately predict outcomes in patients who have a combination of standard and high-risk characteristics [20–23]. Additionally, point-based models are primarily based upon data from interventional clinical trials that may not be representative of Real World NDMM patient populations. The EMPM model here allows differential weighting of the impact of the individual patients and disease-specific risk-factors [24–29].

Patient co-morbidities have been associated with higher mortality in various clinical trials of patients with MM [4, 30–37]. For some NDMM patients, co-morbiditites are both a direct cause of death and places patients at risk for early disease-related mortality by limiting their ability to tolerate therapy [4, 31, 33, 34]. Though the decline the EM to 6.8% reflects the benefit of novel agents and supportive care there are other considerations here. NDMM patients with EM tend to be older and poorer in health with higher rates of co-morbidities (especially diabetes), greater burden of disease, and high-risk features cytogenetics and Stage III disease. The EMPM demonstrates that a lower mobility score, age > 75, history of hypertension, thrombocytopenia, higher ECOG performance status, high ISS disease stage and renal insufficiency were associated with a higher likelihood of EM. Multivariate analysis did not independently find anemia, del(17q) mutation, low self-care score from EQ-SD, hypercalcemia, diabetes and R-ISS score, beta-2 microglobulin and albumin did not predict EM. NDMM patients with EM received more radiation therapy which delayed the initiation of therapy and limited their ability to receive triplet therapy. The EMPM has been validated by bootstrapping for internal cross-validation [38–40]. A high degree of concordance was observed when applying the model using data from patients form the Phase 3 MM-015 trial and the phase 3 FIRST trial despite more rigorous eligibility criteria [41].

This matrix has the potential to be a clinically useful tool for NDMM patients who are at risk for EM and for analyses of specific patient populations, selection of therapy, identification of new targets for treatment and standardized comparisons between trials.

High-quality systematic research to identify patients at risk for EM have not been studied prospectively. The EMPM is the first weight-based model that accounts for both patient and disease-specific risk factors. This model can facilitate early recognition for NDMM patients at high risk for EM to assist physician selection of personalized treatments, avoidance of nephrotoxic agents, monitoring of steroid dosing in diabetic patients, prompt initiation of doublet or triplet therapy and limiting radiation fields when applicable and the use of prophylactic antibiotics. The EMPM can be applied in routine clinical practice and considered in a risk-adaptive approach. Clinical trials of reducing EM patients in NDMM can be designed for new areas of research.

4. Three and five-year overall survival in NDMM

Over the past 60 years, dramatic changes have been made in the treatment of multiple myeloma. These advances have radically altered the disease landscape and prognosis for newly diagnosed patients, turning a previously untreatable illness toward one of a chronic disease [42]. Here we discuss a brief history of treatments and prognostic features in NDMM, the development of novel treatment regimens, and the use of a prediction matrix in 3-year, and 5-year overall survival (OS).

4.1 Historical background of prognostic features

In 1850, Dr. Henry Bence Jones described the first case of myeloma. His patient presented with fatigue, arthralgias, and polyuria. His urine was found to precipitate an unusual protein upon healing, now known as Bence Jones protein. In 1873, Rustizky was found to have multiple osseous masses in a similar patient, giving rise to the name multiple myeloma. In 1889, Kahler presented a large review of the disease, leading it to be called Kahler disease. Over the subsequent several decades, advances in x-ray imaging, microscopy, and electrophoresis allowed for further characterization of the disease. In 1953, immunoelectrophoresis identified excess monoclonal heavy and/or light chains as characteristic for the disease process seen in multiple myeloma [43].

Untreated, NDMM has a median overall survival of two years. In 1958, Blokhin introduced chemotherapy in MM with a mixture of racemic phenylalanine and nitrogen mustards like sacrosine. In 1962, Bergsagel pioneered the use of melphalan and glucocorticoids, creating the combination of melphalan with prednisone (MP), still in use today. However, complete remissions (CR) were rare. In 1983, McElwain and Powles introduced the use of high-dose therapy with melphalan, with CR achieved in a proportion of patients [44]. Those who achieved CR with MP had a median survival of eight years.

Despite the initial advances, the median OS remained at about three years. Remarkably, the current median OS now ranges from 8 to 12 years [45]. However, individual outcomes are varied, with 20% of patients surviving less than 2 years and 40% surviving more than 10 years after diagnosis [46]. Considerable advances in understanding of the pathobiology of multiple myeloma over this time have greatly aided in the ability to select prognostic factors in NDMM. Advances in treatment that have been contributed greatly to survival are reviewed below.

4.2 Prognosis in NDMM

For many years, the factors contributing to the highly variable prognosis in myeloma were unclear. Early on, immunoglobulin isotype was shown to play a role in prognosis, with monoclonal 1gA production (21%) associated with a worse prognosis [47]. The degree of plasma cell burden is only an issue in plasma cell leukemia [48, 49].

In 1975, the Durie-Salmon staging system was adopted, stratifying individuals by relative plasma cell burden (anemia), hypercalcemia, number of lytic lesions visible on x-ray, and serum urine M-protein levels [50]. However, the number of lytic lesions on x-ray is observer-dependent and created challenges with respect to enrollment and reproducibility between trials.

Thirty years later in 2005, Griepp and colleagues established the international staging system (ISS), utilizing the beta-2 microglobulin level and albumin level to appropriately risk-stratify patients. The ISS can predict EFS and OS regardless of age, geographic region, study site, standard-dose vs. high-dose therapy (HDT), or the use of novel agents [51].

Discovery of specific cytogenetic abnormalities correlates with prognosis in multiple myeloma and overall survival. Plasma cells typically have a low-proliferative index, and so cytogenetic abnormalities are detected in a small number of patients. Interphase FISH was found to be useful in identifying specific cytogenetic aberrations [52].

4.3 1gH rearrangements

As the heavy chain of the immunoglobulin molecule is constitutively activated on the 14th chromosome within plasma cells, translocations involving the immunoglobulin heavy chain haven been shown to play a strong role in myeloma pathogenesis and occur in up to half of NDMM patients. Among these 1gH translocations, five appear to be recurrent: t(4;14) and t(11;14), t(4;16) and t(14;20) [53]. The translocations t(4;14) and t(11;14) are not the most common abnormalities involving the 1gVH gene in myeloma, each seen in approximately 15% of patients. These translocations lead to overexpression of FGRF3 and BCL2, respectively. T(4;14) is regarded as high-risk abnormality with inferior median OS. t(11;14) and hyperdiploidy have been reported in some studies to predict a more favorable outcome. T(11;14) is observed in 16–24% of MM patients and has specifically gained interest with the use of the novel agent venetoclax, a BCL2 inhibitor. Currently, the use of venetoclax was stopped due to an early signal for increased death in early clinical trials due to a higher rate of infections [54]. A large, US, multicenter prospective observational cohort study did not demonstrate any impact of t(11;14) on PFS, or OS [55]. Further clinical trials investigating its use in myeloma are currently pending. T(14;16) and T(14;20) are relatively rare, seen in approximately 1.5–3% of patients and lead deregulation of the oncogenes c-MAF and MAFAB, respectively. Though a pivotal trial from the Mayo Clinic was suggestive of poor prognostic correlation with the presence of t(14;16), larger series are uncertain [53].

4.4 del (13)

Though commonly seen in association with other cytogenetic abnormalities in NDMM, del(13) alone does not predict poor outcomes. When occurring in MGUS and SMM it does not influence progression to myeloma. The finding has called into question the use of del(13) in NDMM prognostication [56]. However in the presence of concomitant t(4;14) or del17p, poor prognosis is suggested

del(17p).

The loss of the short term arm of chromosome 17, or del(17p), leads to loss of TP53 and appropriate DNA repair. 17p deletions occur in 8–10% of NDMM patients and has remained a poor risk feature not over by current use of novel therapies. Without adequate DNA repair function, the rate of clonal mutagenesis and subsequent treatment resistance rises more rapidly. Del(17p) is acquired at a median of 35.6 months after the time of diagnosis, with a median PFS of 5.4 months after acquisition. Consequently, as compared to non-del(17p) patients, median OS is significantly worse [57, 58].

4.5 Hyperdiploidy and other cytogenetic abnormalities

In recent years, high-throughput genomic studies using SNP or CGH arrays have accelerated our understanding of genetic changes within NDMM. Hyperdiploidy generally confers a more favorable prognosis in NDMM. The presence of certain trisomies, such as trisomy 3 and trisomy 5, may partially abrogate the negative prognostic features of other cytogenetic abnormalities. In contrast, the presence of trisomy 21 may potentiate the effects of negative prognostic features. Recently identified chromosomal abnormalities, such as gain of 1q and loss of 1q have also been shown to predict for poorer outcomes. One univariate analysis identified poorer prognosis with deletions of 1p, 2p, 14q, 16q, and 22q. Conversely, amplifications of chromosome 5, 11, 15 and 19 were associated with improved outcomes [56]. Chromosome 1q gain has become the most important chromosomal gain abnormality. In a recent update, high risk cytogenetics are presently considered to be del(17p), a p53 mutation, t(4;14), t(14;16),or gain 1q [59]. Similar to lymphoma, the presence of any two or three risk factors is considered 'double-hit' or 'triple-hit' myeloma, respectively.

In 2015, with the advent of cytogenetic profiles, a revised version of the ISS (R-ISS) was adopted, incorporating LDH and high-risk cytogenetics of t(4;14), t(14;16), and del(17p) into the scoring system [60, 61]. These objective systems have allowed for more reproducible results and the ability to more accurately compare patients within clinical trials [61].

However, establishment of baseline disease characteristics are critical for long term prognosis [62]. These newer staging systems do not account for several features that have been shown to correlate to long-term outcomes in myeloma, such as the use of novel myeloma therapies, triplet therapy, autologous stem cell transplant, patient performance status, renal function, a history of diabetes, or MRD status.

Novel agents in multiple myeloma have allowed for significant progress in the treatment of newly diagnosed patients, with more than doubling of the average survival with less toxicity [47].

a. Alkylating agents

In the early 1960's melphalan and cyclophosphamide were the first alkylating agents introduced in the treatment of NDMM demonstrated equivalent activity. In 1972, Harley evaluated other alkylating agents in NDMM, with the use of melphalan, carmustine, and cyclophosphamide, melphalan and prednisone. (MP) was established as the gold standard for treatment, paving the way to several decades of comparison against other combinations of agents, including cyclophosphamide, carmustine, vincristine, and adriamycin. Ultimately, combination therapies improved the response rate in NDMM but did not improve OS compared to MP. MP has a response rate of 50–60%, median PFS of 18 months, and an OS of 30–60 months [63]. To date, melphalan and cyclophosphamide remain effective treatment options and are commonly used in autologous stem-cell transplant conditioning. Combination alkylating agent regimens (such as VD-PACE or VDT-PACE) remain typically reserved for more aggressive disease, as in plasma cell leukemia or refractory MM.

b. Glucocorticoids

Glucocorticoids directly induce apoptosis of plasma cells. This is believed to occur via induction of IkB production that negatively regulates NFkB, resulting in downregulation of IL-6 and other pro-inflammatory cytokines, which facilitates apoptosis of the myeloma clones. In the late 1960's prednisone was added to melphalan, but adoption was slowed due to concerns over the known osteoporosis effect of chronic steroid therapy [44]. Since then, glucocorticoids (particularly dexamethasone) have remained a backbone of therapy. Single-agent dexamethasone is no longer advocated in the treatment of NDMM.

c. IMiDs

An international, randomized phase III trial demonstrated that thalidomide with dexamethasone was superior to dexamethasone alone, with an ORR or 63% vs. 46% and a PFS of 14.9 months vs. 6.5 months [59]. FDA approval in the USA in 1998 of Thalidomide was cautiously accepted due to historical concerns regarding the drug-associated phocomelia was displayed in infants 30 years earlier as antiemetic therapy in pregnancy. Thalidomide is used throughout Europe to date in the treatment of myeloma. Lenalidomide was FDA approved in 2005 based upon rate and lower toxicity profile on a retrospective single-institution case–control study of lenalidomide-dexamethasone vs. thalidomide dexamethasone demonstrated lenalidomide was better tolerated, had a higher ORR of 80% vs. 61%, higher VGPR rate 34 vs. 12%, and improved PFS of 27 months vs. 17 months, establishing lenalidomide with dexamethasone as an appropriate induction option [64]. In 2013, pomalidomide, a second-generation IMiD, was developed for use in relapsed/refractory disease. Though shown to have clear activity in NDMM via several immunomodulation pathways, the precise mechanism of action of these agents remain elusive. Irreversible peripheral neuropathy and increased thrombotic risk remain primary side effects of these agents. Prophylaxis with low-dose aspirin daily is adequate prevention.

d. Proteasome inhibitors

The primary function of plasma cells is to produce immunoglobulin, which occurs on a constitutive basis and requires assembly within 26 s proteasome. Excess accrual of protein within the cell creates proteotoxic stress, leading to cell apoptosis and death. As a result, proteasome inhibitors have been shown to have potent efficacy within the treatment of myeloma. Bortezomib, a boron-containing dipeptide, was the first proteasome inhibitor to be introduced for the treatment of multiple-myeloma. Monotherapy bortezomib FDA approval in 2003 demonstrated an ORR of 27% and a 10% CR rate. In combination with dexamethasone, ORR improved to 88% and CR + VGPR rate of 19%, with a 1-year OS of 87% [65]. Other proteasome inhibitors, including carfilzomib and ixazomib, have been developed and are FDA approved in the relapsed-refractory setting.

Emerging novel agents and therapies

e. Within the past 5 years, several agents have become available in the treatment of multiple myeloma. Notable agents, Dartumumab, a monoclonal antibody against CD-38, has displayed promising efficacy. Belantamab mafadotin, an antibody-drug conjugate between the B-cell maturation antigen (BCMA) and MMAF (a chemotherapy payload) was recently FDA approved for relapsed/refractory disease. BCMA CAR-T cell therapy also shows promise in the relapsed/refractory setting. Though not yet approved in NDMM, these agents, along with others, show promise in the treatment of newly-diagnosed and relapsed-refractory patients.

In 2005, OS in NDMM was 4.6 years, increasing to 6.1 years by 2010. Over the past decade, the adoption of immunomodulatory agents and proteasome inhibitors in triplet therapy extended median OS to greater than 7 years. These gains were predominantly driven by triplet therapy in the elderly and by reducing early mortality in the disease [53, 66].

4.6 Triplet therapy

For many years, monotherapy or doublet regimens were commonly used in the treatment of NDMM. However, with the progressive development of the previously discussed treatment options over the past decades, numerous clinical trials have investigated their use in combination in two-, three-, and four-drug regimens in an attempt to achieve deeper reductions in clonal disease burden. Generally, three-drug combinations (i.e., VCD, VRD, VTD) have been shown to derive the highest ORR and VGPR compared with two-drug regimens and remain the standard of care for fit patients prior to autologous stem cell transplantation (SCT). A Southwest Oncology Group trial randomized 525 patients to either RVD or RD and maintained on RD until progression, with the three-drug combination displaying a better median PFS of 43 months vs. 30 months and median OS 75 vs. 64 months (HR 0.7, $p = 0.025$). As part of triplet therapy, lenalidomide, bortezomib, and dexamethasone (RVD) currently remain standard of care for induction. Though the addition of a fourth drug has not yet shown clear benefit to date, its use likely marks the future, with daratumumab-containing regimens appearing promising. Recently, the GRIFFIN trial compared daratumumab with RVD vs. RVD in NDMM and demonstrated that D-RVD significantly improved strict CR rates and MRD-negativity in transplant-eligible patients [67].

4.7 Autologous stem cell transplant

In the early 1980's, high dose therapy (HDT) with melphalan followed by autologous stem cell transplant (SCT) was performed by McElwain on a patient with plasma cell leukemia. This demonstrated some benefit, but initial adoption was limited due to toxicity of the transplantation process. In the late 1980's, Barlogie further investigated the use of SCT and developed the framework for

SCT in the 1980's and 1990's as part of the standard of care for eligible patients following induction. This led to several prospective, randomized clinical trials in the 1990's which demonstrated superior ORR, PFS, and OS in individuals up to age 65, whereas others demonstrated no survival advantage. Today, SCT following induction therapy in eligible patients remains standard of care. Steady advances in SCT outcomes have occurred over the past 30 years, with patients treated in 2014 or later having superior OS and reduced excess risk for MM death. Second stem cell transplantation may be considered in those with progression-free survival (PFS) or more than three years. Similarly models have supported the potential for cure, estimated at 6.3% to 31.3% depending on the year of treatment [55]. Whether novel agents will supplant HDT followed by SCT backed by minimal residual disease (MRD) continues to be explored. Consideration of myeloablative regimens beyond high-dose melphalan is another venue to be explored for increasing and deepening the CR and MRD negative status.

4.8 Solitary plasmacytoma

Solitary plasmacytomas are uncommon and account for only 6% of all plasma cell neoplasms. They are defined as the presence of a single osseous lesion (medullary) or in the soft tissue outside of the bone (extramedullary) without evidence of bone marrow, clonal plasmacytosis, or CRAB criteria. The incidence of solitary plasmacytomas has increased with increased radiographic imaging use over the past thirty years; incidence increased by 10% from 1999 to 2004 as compared to 1992–1998. Patients with less than 10% plasma cells by bone marrow biopsy can be managed with therapies against the solitary lesion alone, typically 40–50 cGy of radiation or surgical excision alone depending on the location. These patients will eventually progress to MM over the subsequent years but have a generally favorable prognosis, with PFS 63% at 10 years. Extramedullary plasmacytoma has an even more favorable prognosis with myeloma-specific death seen in less than one-third of patients. Progression to MM typically occurs within 5 years from initial diagnosis. Features suggestive of high risk for progression include persistent monoclonal protein after treatment of the solitary lesion, detectable clonal plasma cells in the bone marrow, age 40–60 years old, and individuals of African-American descent. Despite the marked difference in long-term prognosis to NDMM, previous staging systems have not accounted for the presence or absence of solitary plasmacytoma at diagnosis [68].

4.9 Performance status

Baseline performance status has long been understood to play a prominent role in prognosis in NDMM, with unfit patients often remaining ineligible for SCT, the use of triplet therapy, and certain novel therapies. Without these therapies, disease control is less common, and outcomes are worsened. Furthermore, clinical trials commonly select for fit patients (typically.

ECOG 0–1), reducing the generalization of data to community setting, where less fit patients are encountered with greater frequency.

4.10 Renal function

Baseline renal function in NDMM patients is an essential part of long-term prognosis. Impaired renal function at baseline limits the usage of novel agents that can be administered, as many are renally cleared. Persistent renal dysfunction limits what therapeutic options are available and thus long-term outcomes are worse [69]. As cyclophosphamide is hepatically cleared, cyclophosphamide, bortezomib, and dexamethasone remains standard induction regimen in individuals with compromised renal function. Melphalan, which is cleared through spontaneous hydrolysis, is another renal-independent therapeutic option. Previous risk-stratification systems have not addressed this conundrum with renal dysfunction.

4.11 Diabetes

Comorbidities present in NDMM patients play a strong role in what therapies may be available [70]. Diabetes mellitus, owing to concomitant progressive renal dysfunction and peripheral neuropathy, may limit the use or dose of certain novel therapies. Both IMiDs and proteasome inhibitors may worsen peripheral neuropathy, potentially limiting the dose able to be given or as a class altogether depending on the severity of neuropathy. Diabetic nephropathy poses similar limitations.

4.12 Minimal residual disease

In every NDMM patient, there are an average of 3 to 5 clones present. These clones undergo mutations at varying degrees throughout the treatment course, with progression of disease presenting expansion of resistant clones over time. As a result, multiple myeloma is not considered to be a curable disease, and so an evolving treatment aim has been for maximal disease burden reduction [71]. The ability to reduce disease burden beneath the threshold of detection, known as minimal residual disease (MRD), has been shown to be an important prognostic indicator for survival and long-term outcomes. MRD has traditionally been detected by flow cytometry (sensitive to 10^4 cells) and next generation sequencing (NGS) (sensitive 10^6 cells). An evolving consensus is that achieving MRD-negative status at the time of induction therapy should be the goal of therapy. Though not-yet involved in staging systems, MRD-focused treatment assessments are becoming increasingly important with time [72].

4.13 Next-generation sequencing

NGS when it comes to FISH (seq-FISH) has improved sensitivity and similar specifically relative to clinical FISH studies and appears to identify a higher number of high-risk NDMM patients. These studies are currently ongoing to incorporate into routine staging systems [4, 29].

4.14 Predictive models in NDMM

Multiple advances in long-term survival have been made over time, with the potential for cure by some models. Heterogeneity of prognostic factors in multiple myeloma makes accurate prognostication difficult on an individual level. As a result, the use of prediction matrix and prognostic tools have aided our ability to assess overall survival. Furthermore, owing to the selection bias present within clinical trials populations, survival estimates derived from clinical trials limit the applicability to all "Real World" patients. The CONNECT® registry was created as a prognostic model for OS in an unselected community and academic setting [66]. Prognostic models should take into account myeloma biology, patient comorbidities and include performance status and mobility assessment [73]. Next Gen Sequencing will offer a more comprehensive approach to treatment and the goal of a MRD negative NDMM patient.

Author details

Howard R. Terebelo[1,2]* and Leo Reap[1,2]

1 Ascension Providence Hospital, Department of Hematology and Oncology, Southfield, Michigan, USA

2 Michigan State University, East Lansing, Michigan, USA

*Address all correspondence to: hiccup@comcast.net

References

[1] Murakami H, Hayashi K, Hatsumi N, et al. Risk factors for early death in patients undergoing treatment for multiple myeloma. Ann Hematol. 2001;80:452-455. https://doi.org/10.1007/s002770100330

[2] Kastritis E, Terpos E, Roussou M, et al. Very early death (< 2 months) in myeloma is associated with advanced age, poor performance status and reduced use of novel agents, while early death within 12 months is associated with high risk features of both the disease and the patient. Blood. 2013;122:[abstract 3195]. https://doi.org/10.1182/blood.V122.21.3195.3195

[3] Biran N, Jagannath S, Chari A. Risk stratification in multiple myeloma, part 1: characterization of high-risk disease. Clin Adv Hematol Oncol. 2013;11:489-503. PMID: 24518420.

[4] Larocca A, Bringhen S, Petrucci M, et al. Early mortality in elderly newly diagnosed multiple myeloma patients treated with novel agents: a pooled analysis of two large randomized phase III trials. Haematologica. 2015;100:[abstract P270].

[5] Augustson BM, Begum G, Dunn JA, et al. Early mortality after diagnosis of multiple myeloma: analysis of patients entered onto the United Kingdom Medical Research Council trials between 1980 and 2002–Medical Research Council Adult Leukaemia Working Party. J Clin Oncol. 2005;23:9219-9226. https://doi/10.1200/JCO.2005.03.2086

[6] Rana V, Srivastava G, Hayman SR, et al. Factors predicting early mortality in patients with newly diagnosed multiple myeloma. Blood. 2011;118:[abstract 3981]. https://doi.org/10.1182/blood.V118.21.3981.3981

[7] Moreau P, Cavo M, Sonneveld P, et al. Combination of International Scoring System 3, high lactate dehydrogenase, and t(4;14) and/or del(17p) identifies patients with multiple myeloma (MM) treated with front-line autologous stem-cell transplantation at high risk of early MM progression-related death. J Clin Oncol. 2014;32:2173-2180. https://doi.org/10.1200/JCO.2013.53.0329

[8] Conroy RM, Pyorala K, Fitzgerald AP, et al. Estimation of ten-year risk of fatal cardiovascular disease in Europe: the SCORE project. Eur Heart J. 2003;24:987-1003. https://doi.org/10.1016/s0195-668x(03)00114-3

[9] Vastesaeger N, Xu S, Aletaha D, et al. A pilot risk model for the prediction of rapid radiographic progression in rheumatoid arthritis. Rheumatology. 2009;48:1114-1121. https://doi.org/10.1093/rheumatology/kep155

[10] Appelbaum FR, Gundacker H, Head DR, et al. Age and acute myeloid leukemia. Blood. 2006;107:3481-3485. https://doi.org/10.1182/blood-2005-09-3724

[11] Rosenwald A, Wright G, Chan WC, et al. The use of molecular profiling to predict survival after chemotherapy for diffuse large-B-cell lymphoma. N Engl J Med. 2002;346:1937-1947. https://doi.org/101056/NEJMoa012914

[12] Lin C, Itti E, Haioun C, et al. Early 18F-FDG PET for prediction of prognosis in patients with diffuse large B-cell lymphoma: SUV-based assessment versus visual analysis. J Nucl Med. 2007;48:1626-1632. https://doi.org/10.2967/jnumed.107.042093

[13] Rifkin RM, Abonour R, Terebelo H, et al. Connect MM registry: the importance of establishing baseline disease characteristics. Clin Lymphoma Myeloma Leuk. 2015;15:368-376. https://doi.org/10.1016/j.clml.2014.12.002

[14] Levine MN, Julian JA. Registries that show efficacy: good, but not good enough. J Clin Oncol. 2008;26:5316-5319. https://doi.org/10.1200.JCO.2008.18.3996

[15] Gliklich R, Dreyer N, Leavy M and eds. Registries for Evaluating Patient Outcomes: A User's Guide. Third edition. Two volumes. (Prepared by the Outcome DEcIDE Center [Outcome Sciences, Inc., a Quintiles company] under Contract No. 290 2005 00351 TO7.) AHRQ Publication No. 13(14)-EHC111. Rockville, MD: Agency for Healthcare Research and Quality. April 2014. http://www.effectivehealthcare.ahrq.gov/registries-guide-3.cfm.

[16] Yoshida K, Radner H, Kavanaugh A, et al. Use of data from multiple registries in studying biologic discontinuation: challenges and opportunities. Clin Exp Rheumatol. 2013;31:S28–S32. PMID24129133

[17] Kumar SK, Dispenzieri A, Lacy MQ, et al. Continued improvement in survival in multiple myeloma: changes in early mortality and outcomes in older patients. Leukemia. 2014;28:1122-1128. https://doi.org/10.1038/leu.2013.313

[18] Beksac M, Haznedar R, Firatli-Tuglular T, et al. Addition of thalidomide to oral melphalan/prednisone in patients with multiple myeloma not eligible for transplantation: results of a randomized trial from the Turkish Myeloma Study Group. Eur J Haematol. 2011;86:16-22. https://doi.org/10.1111/j-1600-0609.2010.01524.x

[19] Gonsalves WI, Godby K, Kumar SK, Costa LJ. Limiting early mortality: do's and don'ts in the management of patients with newly diagnosed multiple myeloma. Am J Hematol. 2016;91:101-108. https://doi.org/10.1002/ajh.24129

[20] Palumbo A, Avet-Loiseau H, Oliva S, et al. Revised International Staging System for multiple myeloma: a report from International Myeloma Working Group. J Clin Oncol. 2015;33:2863-2869. https://doi.org/10.1200/JCO.2015.61.2267

[21] Ozaki S, Harada T, Saitoh T, et al. Survival of multiple myeloma patients aged 65-70 years in the era of novel agents and autologous stem cell transplantation. A multicenter retrospective collaborative study of the Japanese Society of Myeloma and the European Myeloma Network. Acta Haematol. 2014;132:211-219. https://doi.org/10.1159/000357394

[22] Palumbo A, Bringhen S, Mateos MV, et al. Geriatric assessment predicts survival and toxicities in elderly myeloma: an International Myeloma Working Group report. Blood. 2015;125:2068-2074. https://doi.org/10.1182/blod-2014-12-615187

[23] Mehta J, Cavo M, Singhal S. How I treat elderly patients with myeloma. Blood. 2010;116:2215-2223. https://doi.org/10.1182/blood-2009-10-163329

[24] Oken MM, Creech RH, Tormey DC, et al. Toxicity and response criteria of the Eastern Cooperative Oncology Group. Am J Clin Oncol. 1982;5:649-655. PMID: 7165009

[25] European Society for Medical Oncology (ESMO) . Performance scales: Karnofsky & ECOG scores. http://oncologypro.esmo.org/Guidelines-Practice/Practice-Tools/Performance-Scales. Accessed October 27, 2015. PMID7165009

[26] Mohty M, Cavo, Fink, L et al. Understanding mortality in multiple myeloma: findings of a European chart review. Eur J Haematol.2019; 103(20:107-115 https://doi.org/10.1111/ejh.13264

[27] Xia J, Wang L, Zhou X, et al. Early mortality in elderly patients undergoing

treatment for multiple myeloma in real-world practice. Journal of International Medical Research. https://doi.org/0.1177/0300060518757640

[28] Bringhen S, Offidani M, Palmieri S, et al. Early mortality in myeloma patients treated with first-generation novel agents thalidomide, lenalidomide, bortezomib at diagnosis: a pooled analysis. Critical Reviews in Oncology/Hematology. Vol 130; Oct 2018:27-35 https://doi.org/10.1016/j.critrevonc.2018.07.003

[29] Goldsmith S, Fiala M, Dukeman, J et al. Next generation sequencing-based validation of the revised international staging system for multiple myeloma: an analysis of MMRF CoMMpass study. Clin Lymphoma Myeloma Leuk. 2019 May 19 (5):285-289 https://doi.org/10.1016/j.clml.2019.01.003

[30] Costa LJ, Gonsalves WI, Kumar SK. Early mortality in multiple myeloma. Leukemia. 2015;29:1616-1618. https://doi.org/10.1038/leu.2015.33

[31] Dimopoulos MA, Delimpasi S, Katodritou E, et al. Significant improvement in the survival of patients with multiple myeloma presenting with severe renal impairment after the introduction of novel agents. Ann Oncol. 2014;25:195-200. https://doi.org/10.1093/annonc/mdt483

[32] Zomas A, Terpos E, Kastritis E, et al. Hypercalcemia remains an adverse prognostic factor for newly diagnosed patients with symptomatic multiple myeloma in the era of novel anti-myeloma therapies, independently of age, ISS stage and treatment type: an analysis of 2129 patients. Blood. 2014;124:[abstract 2113]. https://doi.org/10.1182/blood.V124.21.2113.2113

[33] Kumar S. Risk of early death in multiple myeloma. Clin Adv Hematol Oncol. 2012;10:172-174. PMID:22402425

[34] Holmstrom MO, Gimsing P, Abildgaard N, et al. Causes of early death in multiple myeloma patients who are ineligible for high-dose therapy with hematopoietic stem cell support: a study based on the nationwide Danish Myeloma Database. Am J Hematol. 2015;90:E73–E74. https://doi.org/10.1002/ajh.23932

[35] Mey UJM, Leitner C, Driessen C, et al. Improved survival of older patients with multiple myeloma in the era of novel agents. Hematol Oncol. 2016;34:217-223. https://doi.org/10.1002/hon.2205

[36] Chng WJ, Dispenzieri A, Chim CS, et al. IMWG consensus on risk stratification in multiple myeloma. Leukemia. 2014;28:269-277. https://doi.org/10.1038/leu.2013.247

[37] Mikhael JR, Dingli D, Roy V, et al. Management of newly diagnosed symptomatic multiple myeloma: updated Mayo Stratification of Myeloma and Risk-Adapted Therapy (mSMART) consensus guidelines 2013. Mayo Clin Proc. 2013;88:360-376. https://doi.org/10.1016/j.mayocp.2013.01.019

[38] Bernaards CA, Belin TR, Schafer JL. Robustness of a multivariate normal approximation for imputation of incomplete binary data. Stat Med. 2007;26:1368-1382. https://doi.org/10.1002/sim.2619

[39] Steyerberg EW, Vickers AJ, Cook NR, et al. Assessing the performance of prediction models: a framework for some traditional and novel measures. Epidemiology. 2010;21:128-138. https://doi.org/10.1097/EDE.0b013e3181c30fb2

[40] Palumbo A, Hajek R, Delforge M, et al. Continuous lenalidomide treatment for newly diagnosed multiple myeloma. N Engl J Med. 2012;366:1759-1769. https://doi.org/10.1056/NEJMoa1112704

[41] Benboubker L, Dimopoulos MA, Dispenzieri A, et al. Lenalidomide and dexamethasone in transplant-ineligible patients with myeloma. N Engl J Med. 2014;371:906-917. https://doi.org/10.1056/NEJMoa1402551

[42] Kyle RA, Rajkumar SV. Multiple Myeloma. Blood. 2008;111(6):2962-2972. https://doi.org/10.1182/blood-2007-10-078022

[43] Kyle RA, Steensma DP. History of Multiple Myeloma. Multiple Myeloma. 2011:3-23. https://doi.org/10.1007/978-3-540-85772-3_1

[44] Ribatti D. A historical perspective on milestones in multiple myeloma research. European Journal of Haematology. 2017;100(3):221-228. doi:10.1111/ejh. 13003

[45] Nandakumar B, Binder M, Dispenzieri A, et al. Continued improvement in survival in multiple myeloma (MM) including high-risk patients. Journal of Clinical Oncology. 2019;37(15_suppl):8039-8039. https://doi.org/10.1200/jco.2019.37.15_suppl.8039

[46] Jagannath S, Rifkin RM, Gasparetto CJ, et al. Treatment Journeys of Patients With Newly Diagnosed Multiple Myeloma (NDMM): Results From the Connect MM Registry. Clinical Lymphoma Myeloma and Leukemia. 2020;20(5):272-276. Doi:10.1016/j.clml.2019.10.002 https://doi.org/10.1016/j.clml.2019.10.002

[47] Nair B, Waheed S, Szymonifka J, Shaughnessy Jr JD, Crowley J, Barlogie B. Immunoglobulin isotypes in multiple myeloma: laboratory correlates and prognostic implications in total therapy protocols. British Journal of Haematology. 2009;145(1):134-137. https://doi.org/10.1111/j.1365-2141.2008.07547.x

[48] Lopez A, Abrisqueta P. Plasmablastic lymphoma: current perspectives. Blood and Lymphatic Cancer: Targets and Therapy. 2018;Volume 8:63-70. https://doi.org/10.2147/blctts.s142814

[49] Sher T, Miller KC, Deeb G, Lee K, Chanan-Khan A. Plasma cell leukemia and other aggressive plasma cell malignancies. British Journal of Haematology. 2010; 150(4):418-427. https://doi.org/10.1111/j.1354-2141.2010.08157.x

[50] Durie, BGM and Salmon, SE (1975), A clinical staging system for multiple myeloma correlation of measured myeloma cell mass with presenting clinical features, response to treatment, and survival. Cancer, 36: 842-854. https://doi.org/10.1002/1097-0142(197509)B36:3>3.0CO;2-U

[51] Greipp PR, San Miguel J, Durie BG, Crowley JJ, Barlogie B, Bladé J, Boccadoro M, Child JA, Avet-Loiseau H, Kyle RA, Lahuerta JJ, Ludwig H, MorganG,PowlesR,ShimizuK,ShustikC, Sonneveld P, Tosi P, Turesson I, Westin J. International staging system for multiple myeloma. J Clin Oncol. 2005 May 20;23(15):3412-20. https://doi.org/10.1200/JCO.2005.04.242. Epub 2005 Apr 4. Erratum in JCO. 2005 Sep 1;23(25):6281. Harousseau, Jean-Luc [corrected to Avet-Loiseau, Herve]. PMID:15809451

[52] Dascalescu CM, Callanan M, Chauvet M, et al. Interphase FISH: a rapid method for detecting malignant plasma cells in multiple myeloma patients submitted to autologous transplantation. Bone Marrow Transplantation. 1999;23(7):687-694. https://doi.org/10.1038/sj.bmt.1701626

[53] Lee HC, Ailawadhi S, Gasparetto C, et al. Treatment Patterns and Outcomes in Elderly Patients with Newly Diagnosed Multiple Myeloma: Results from the Connect ® MM Registry. Blood. 2019;134(Supplement_1):3129-3129.

https://doi.org/10.1182/blood-2019-126205

[54] Kumar SK, Harrison SJ, Cavo M. et al. Venetoclax or placebo in combination with bortezomib and dexamethasone in patients with relapsed or refractory multiple myeloma (BELLINI): a randomised, double-blind, multicentre, phase 3 trial. The Lancet Oncology. 2020. https://doi.org/10.1016/s1470-2045(20)30525-8

[55] Nishimura KK, Barlogie B, van Rhee F, et al., Long-term outcomes after autologous stem cell transplantation for multiple myeloma. Blood Advances. 2020;4(2):422-431. https://doi.org/10.1182/bloodadvances.2019000524

[56] Sonneveld P, Avet-Loiseau H, Lonial S, et al. Treatment of multiple myeloma with high-risk cytogenetics: a consensus of the International Myeloma Working Group. Blood. 2016;127(4):2955-2962. https://doi.org/10.1182/blood-2016-01-631200

[57] Durie BGM, Hoering A, Sexton R, et al. Longer term follow-up of the randomized phase III trial SWOG S0777: bortezomib, lenalidomide and dexamethasone vs. lenalidomide and dexamethasone in patients (Pts) with previously untreated multiple myeloma without an intent for immediate autologous stem cell transplant (ASCT). Blood Cancer Journal. 2020;10(5). https://doi.org/10.1038/s41408-020-0311-8

[58] Lakshman A, Painly U, Rajkumar SV, et al. Impact of acquired del(17p) in multiple myeloma. Blood Advances. 2019;3(13):1930-1938. https://doi.org/10.1182/bloodadvances.2018028530

[59] Rajkumar SV, Blood E, Vesole D, Fonseca R, Greipp PR. Phase III Clinical Trial of Thalidomide Plus Dexamethasone Compared With Dexamethasone Alone in Newly Diagnosed Multiple Myeloma: A Clinical Trial Coordinated by the Eastern Cooperative Oncology Group. Journal of Clinical Oncology. 2006;24(3):431-436. https://doi.org/10.1200/jco.2005.03.0221

[60] Palumbo A, Avet-Loiseau H, Olivia S, et al. Revised International Staging System for Multiple Myeloma: A Report From International Myeloma Working Group. Journal of Clinical Oncology. 2015;33(26):2863-2869. https://doi.org/10.1200/jco.201.61.2267

[61] Abdalla N, Rajkumar SV, Greipp P, et al. Cytogenetics abnormalities in multiple myeloma: association with disease characteristics and treatment response. Blood Cancer Journal. 2020;10(8).https://doi.org/10.1038/s41408-020-00348-5

[62] Rifkin RM, Abonour R, Terebelo H, et al. Connect MM Registry: The Importance of Establishing Baseline Disease Characteristics. Clinical Lymphoma Myeloma and Leukemia. 2015;15(6):368-376. https://doi.org/10.1016/j.clm.2014.12.002

[63] Zweegman S, van der Holt B, Mellqvist U-H, et al. Melphalan, prednisone, and lenalidomide versus melphalan, prednisone, and thalidomide in untreated multiple myeloma. Blood. 2016;127(9):1109-1116. https://doi.org/10.1182/blood-2015-11-679415

[64] Gay F, Hayman SR, Lacy MQ, et al. Lenalidomide plus dexamethasone versus thalidomide plus dexamethasone in newly diagnosed multiple myeloma: a comparative analysis of 114 patients. Blood. 2010;115(7):1343-1350. https://doi.org/10.1182/blood-2009-08-239046

[65] Moreau P, Richardson PG, Cavo M, et al. Proteasome inhibitors in multiple myeloma: 10 years later. Blood. 2012;120(5):947-959. https://doi.org/10.1182/blood-2012-04-403733

[66] Terebelo HR, Abonour R, Gaspretto CJ, et al. Development of a prognostic model for overall survival in multiple myeloma using the Connect ® MM Patient Registry. British Journal of Haematology. 2019; 187(5):602-614. doi:10.111/bjh. 16139 https://doi.org/10.111/bjh.16139

[67] Voorhees PM, Kaufman JL, Laubach J, et al. Daratumumab, lenalidomide, bortezomib, and dexamethasone for transplant-eligible newly diagnosed multiple myeloma: the GRIFFIN trial. Blood. 2020;136(8): 936-945. https://doi.org/10.1182/blood.2020005288

[68] Pham A, Mahindra A. Solitary Plasmacytoma: a Review of Diagnosis and Management. Current Hematologic Malignancy Reports. 2019;14(2):63-69. https://doi.org/10.1007/s11899-019-00499-8

[69] Gregersen H, Vangsted AJ, Abildgaard N, et al. The impact of comorbidity on mortality in multiple myeloma: a Danish nationwide population-based study. Cancer Medicine. 2017;6(7):1807-1816. https://doi.org/10.1002/cam4.1128

[70] Chen YJ, De AP, Cong Z, Aggarwal SK, Wade RL. Demographic and Comorbidity Characteristics of Newly Diagnosed Multiple Myeloma Patients in the United States: A Real World Data Analysis. Blood. 2014;124(21):1301-1301 https://doi.org/10.1182/blood.V124.21.1301.1301

[71] Magrangeas F, Avet-Loiseau H, Gouraud W. et al. Minor clone provides a reservoir for relapse in multiple myeloma. Leukemia. 2012;27(2): 473-481. https://doi.org/10.1038/leu.2012.226

[72] Kostopoulos IV, Ntanasis-Stathopoulos I, Gavriatopoulou M, Tsitsilonis OE, Terpos E. Minimal Residual Disease in Multiple Myeloma: Current Landscape and Future Applications with Immunotherapeutic Approaches. Frontiers in Oncology. 2020;10. https://doi.org/10.3389/fonc.2020.00860

[73] Terebelo H, Srinivasan S, Narang M, et al. Recognition of early mortality in multiple myeloma by a prediction matrix. American Journal of Hematology. 2017;92(9):915-923. https://doi.org/10.1002/ajh.24796

Chapter 3

Treatment Approaches of Multiple Myeloma

Minyahil Alebachew Woldu, Atalay Mulu Fentie and Tamrat Assefa Tadesse

Abstract

Multiple Myeloma (MM) is the most common malignant neoplasm of plasma cells that accumulate in bone marrow, leading to bone destruction and marrow failure. Clinical investigation of MM requires the evaluation of bone marrow for plasma cell infiltration, and detection and quantification of monoclonal protein in the serum or urine, and evidence for end-organ damage (i.e., hypercalcemia, renal insufficiency, anemia, or bone lesions). The overall goal of treatment of MM is to improve survival. The treatment landscape and clinical outcome of MM have changed in the last two decades, with an improved median survival of 8–10 years. Management of MM involves induction, consolidation, and maintenance therapy. Currently, Autologous stem cell transplant (ASCT) is considered as the standard care of treatment for newly diagnosed fit MM patients. Multiple combinations of proteasome inhibitors (PIs) and immunomodulatory drugs (IMIDs) such as Thalidomide, lenalidomide, and pomalidomide have been under evaluation in ASCT-eligible and ineligible settings, and studies are still ongoing. For patients with ASCT-eligible newly diagnosed MM, induction therapy with triple drugs should contain an IMiD, a PI, and a corticosteroid, usually lenalidomide-bortezomib-dexamethasone. For ASCT-ineligible patients on lenalidomide with dexamethasone (Rd), with addition of bortezomib or daratumumab can be considered.

Keywords: Pharmacotherapy of Multiple Myeloma, Standard Treatment of Multiple Myeloma, Advances in Management of Multiple Myeloma

1. Introduction

Multiple Myeloma (MM) is the most common type of plasma cells cancer that mount up from bone marrows, and leads to osteodysfunction and marrow failure [1, 2]. It is second to non-Hodgkin lymphoma as the most common hematologic malignancy [3]. Majority of the MM patients who develop Monoclonal Gammopathy of Undetermined Significance (MGUS) are initially pass through the stage of asymptomatic pre-malignancy [4, 5]. The conversion of MGUS to MM is around 1% per annum, and the more advanced form of pre-malignant stage termed as Smoldering (or indolent) MM (SMM) can also be seen in some patients, that has a progression rate of 10% per annum over the first 5 years of diagnosis, 3% per year over the following 5 years, and 1.5% per year thereafter [4–6].

The European Myeloma Network (EMN) provides recommendations for the management of the most common complications of MM. The whole body low-dose computed tomography (LDCT) is now considered as novel in detecting lytic lesions, and more sensitive than conventional radiography in depicting osteolytic disease as per the recommendations of the EMN [7, 8].

The treatment landscape and clinical outcome of MM have changed in the last two decades, with an improved median survival of 8–10 years [9]. The initial impact seen with the introduction of three drugs, thalidomide, bortezomib, and lenalidomide [10]. Multiple combinations of proteasome inhibitors (PIs) like bortezomib, carfilzomib, and ixazomib; immunomodulatory drugs (IMIDs) such as Thalidomide, lenalidomide, and pomalidomide; corticosteroids (Cs) such as dexamethasone, prednisone; monoclonal antibodies (MAs) like Daratumumab and isatuximab; and alkylating agents such as melphalan, cyclophosphamide have been tried and evaluated in the transplant and non-transplant settings, and studies are still ongoing [9]. The approval of carfilzomib, pomalidomide, panobinostat, ixazomib, elotuzumab, and daratumumab by the Food and Drug Administration (FDA) for the treatment of relapsed multiple myeloma, in the last five years is an step closer to radical cure [10].

2. Diagnosis

Clinical investigation of MM requires the evaluation of bone marrow for plasma cell infiltration, and detection and quantification of monoclonal protein in the serum or urine, and evidence for end-organ damage (i.e., hypercalcemia, renal insufficiency, anemia, or bone lesions) [11, 12]. This can be done by grouping the different diagnostic and prognostic factors measurable parameters, such as protein analysis, morphology, immunophenotyping, genetics and cytogenetics, and imaging techniques (i.e., MRI, PET/CT) [11].

2.1 Staging in myeloma

According to the International Myeloma Working Group (IMWG) criteria, the diagnosis of MM requires a 10% or more clonal plasma cells infiltration of the bone marrow and/or a biopsy proven plasmacytoma plus any one or more of the myeloma defining events (MDE) which include end-organ damage, characterized by hypercalcemia, renal insufficiency, anemia, or bone lesions which attributable to the underlying plasma-cell disorder; bone marrow clonal plasma cells ≥60%; serum involved to uninvolved free light chain (FLC) ratio ≥ 100 (provided involved FLC level is ≥100 mg/L); or magnetic resonance imaging (MRI) result of more than 1 focal lesion (5 mm or more in size) [10].

2.2 Revised international staging system for myeloma

The following staging is as per the IMWG [13].

1. **Stage I** MM patient will have (all of the following): normal serum lactate dehydrogenase level and without high cytogenetic features; and they will have serum beta-2-microglobulin of <3.5 mg/L and serum albumin level > 3.5 g/dL.

2. **Stage II** patient will have neither stage I or III criteria

3. **Stage III** MM patient will have serum beta-2-microglobulin >5.5 mg/L; and either high risk cytogenetics [t(4;14), t(14;16), or del(17p)] or an elevated serum lactate dehydrogenase level.

Regimen	Usual dosing schedule[a]
Lenalidomide-dexamethasone (Rd)	Lenalidomide 25 mg oral days 1–21 every 28 days Dexamethasone 40 mg oral days 1, 8, 15, 22 every 28 days Repeated every 4 wk
Thalidomide-dexamethasone (Td)[b]	Thalidomide 200 mg oral days 1–28 Dexamethasone 40 mg oral days 1, 8, 15, 22 Repeated every 4 weeks
Bortezomib-melphalan-prednisone (VMP)[b]	Bortezomib 1.3 mg/m^2 subcutaneous days 1, 8, 15, 22 Melphalan 9 mg/m^2 oral days 1–4 Prednisone 60 mg/m^2 oral days 1 to 4 Repeated every 35 days
Pomalidomide-dexamethasone (Pom/Dex)	Pomalidomide 4 mg days 1–21 Dexamethasone 40 mg oral on days on days 1, 8, 15, 22 Repeated every 4 wk
Bortezomib-Cyclophosphamide-Dexamethasoneb (VCd or CyBord)	Cyclophosphamide 300 mg/m^2 orally on days 1, 8, 15, and 22 Bortezomib 1.3 mg/m^2 subcutaneous on days 1, 8, 15, 22 Dexamethasone 40 mg oral on days on days 1, 8, 15, 22 Repeated every 4 weeks[c]
Bortezomib-thalidomide-dexamethasone (VTd)[b]	Bortezomib 1.3 mg/m^2 subcutaneous days 1, 8, 15, 22 Thalidomide 100–200 mg oral days 1–21 Dexamethasone 20 mg oral on day of and day after bortezomib (or 40 mg days 1, 8, 15, 22) Repeated every 4 weeks 3 4 cycles as pretransplant induction therapy
Carfilzomib-Cyclophosphamide-Dexamethasone (KCd)	Carfilzomib 20 mg/m^2 (days 1 and 2 of Cycle 1) and 27 mg/m^2 (subsequent doses) intravenously on days 1, 2, 8, 9, 15, 16 Cyclophosphamide 300 mg/m^2 orally on days 1, 8, 15 Dexamethasone 40 mg oral on days on days 1, 8, 15, 22 Repeated every 4 weeks
Bortezomib-Lenalidomide-Dexamethasone (VRd)[b]	Bortezomib 1.3 mg/m^2 subcutaneous days 1, 8, 15 Lenalidomide 25 mg oral days 1–14 Dexamethasone 20 mg oral on day of and day after bortezomib (or 40 mg days 1, 8, 15, 22) Repeated every 3 weeks[d]
Carfilzomib-Lenalidomide-Dexamethasone (KRd)[e]	Carfilzomib 20 mg/m^2 (days 1 and 2 of Cycle 1) and 27 mg/ m^2 (subsequent doses) intravenously on days 1, 2, 8, 9, 15, 16 Lenalidomide 25 mg oral days 1–21 Dexamethasone 40 mg oral days 1, 8, 15, 22 Repeated every 4 weeks
Carfilzomib-Pomalidomide-Dexamethasone (KPd)[e]	Carfilzomib 20 mg/m^2 (days 1 and 2 of Cycle 1) and 27 mg/ m^2 (subsequent cycles) intravenously on days 1, 2, 8, 9, 15, 16 Pomalidomide 4 mg oral on days 1–21 Dexamethasone 40 mg oral on days on days 1, 8, 15, 22 Repeated every 4 weeks
Daratumumab-Lenalidomide-Dexamethasone (DRd)	Daratumumab 16 mg/ kg intravenously weekly × 8 weeks, and then every 2 weeks for 4 months, and then once monthly Lenalidomide 25 mg oral days 1–21 Dexamethasone 40 mg intravenous days 1, 8, 15, 22 (given oral on days when no daratumumab is being administered) Lenalidomide-Dexamethasone repeated in usual schedule every 4 weeks
Daratumumab-Bortezomib-Dexamethasone (DVd)[b]	Daratumumab 16 mg/ kg intravenously weekly × 8 weeks, and then every 2 weeks for 4 months, and then once monthly Bortezomib 1.3 mg/m^2 subcutaneous on days 1, 8, 15, 22 Dexamethasone 40 mg intravenous days 1, 8, 15, 22 (given oral on days when no daratumumab is being administered) Bortezomib-Dexamethasone repeated in usual schedule every 4 weeks

Regimen	Usual dosing schedule[a]
Daratumumab-Pomalidomide-Dexamethasone (DPd)	Daratumumab 16 mg/kg intravenously weekly 3 8 weeks, and then every 2 weeks for 4 months, and then once monthly Pomalidomide 4 mg oral on days 1–21 Dexamethasone 40 mg intravenous days 1, 8, 15, 22 (given oral on days when no daratumumab is being administered) Repeated every 4 weeks
Elotuzumab-Lenalidomide-Dexamethasone (ERd)	10 mg/ kg intravenously weekly × 8 weeks, and then every 2 weeks Lenalidomide 25 mg oral days 1–21 Dexamethasone per prescribing information Lenalidomide-Dexamethasone repeated in usual schedule every 4 weeks
Ixazomib-Lenalidomide-Dexamethasone (IRd)	Ixazomib 4 mg oral days 1, 8, 15 Lenalidomide 25 mg oral days 1–21 Dexamethasone 40 mg oral days 1, 8, 15, 22 Repeated every 4 weeks
Panobinostat-Bortezomib[b]	Panobinostat 20 mg oral three times a week 3 2 weeks Bortezomib 1.3 mg/m^2 subcutaneous days 1, 8, 15 Repeated every 3 weeks

[a]*All doses need to be adjusted for performance status, renal function, blood counts, and other toxicities.*
[b]*Doses of dexamethasone and/or bortezomib reduced based on other data showing lower toxicity and similar efficacy with reduced doses; subcutaneous route of administration of bortezomib preferred based on data showing lower toxicity and similar efficacy compared to intravenous administration.*
[c]*The day 22 dose of all 3 drugs is omitted if counts are low, or after initial response to improve tolerability, or when the regimen is used as maintenance therapy; When used as maintenance therapy for high risk patients, further delays can be instituted between cycles.*
[d]*Omit day 15 dose if counts are low or when the regimen is used as maintenance therapy; When used as maintenance therapy for high risk patients, lenalidomide dose may be decreased to 10–15 mg per day, and delays can be instituted between cycles as done in total therapy protocols.*
[e]*Carfilzomib can also considered in a once a week schedule of 70 mg/m^2 on days 1, 8 and 15 every 28 days (cycle 1, day 1 should be 20 mg/m^2); Day 8, 9 doses of carfilzomib can be omitted in maintenance phase of therapy after a good response to improve tolerability; KCd dosing lowered from that used in the initial trial which was conducted in newly diagnosed patients.*

Table 1.
Major treatment regimens in multiple myeloma [9, 10].

Different ranges of regimens have been developed to retard progression of disease using potentially effective in controlling and promising for survival. The most commonly used drug combinations are listed in **Table 1**.

2.3 Symptomatic versus asymptomatic myeloma

Urgent management of indolent myeloma is not recommended at the present time; rather treatment should be considered in all symptomatic patients with an active myeloma criteria (the CRAB criteria) (hypercalcaemia >11.0 mg/dl), creatinine >2.0 mg/ml, anemia (Hb < 10 mg/dL), active bone lesions), [9].

3. Goal of treatment

The overall goal of treatment of MM is to improve survival [14, 15]. A complete response (CR) has been observed only in few patients with conventional chemotherapy regimens. The use of high-dose therapy followed by ASCT and the advent of novel therapies, such as thalidomide, lenalidomide, and bortezomib gained much promises [14, 15], and with such treatment many patients are gaining the much needed improvement and CR. Studies reported that the success of CR correlates with survival, and hence the role of CR as an endpoint in myeloma therapy is becoming prominence. It should also be noted that the benefit of CR is not the same with all treatment regimens [15, 16]. Emerging evidence with novel medications showed that continued treatment has resulted in prolong CR and improved response [16].

4. Management of newly diagnosed cases

Currently, for fit newly diagnosed MM patients (NDMM), autologous stem cell transplant (ASCT) considered as the standard care of treatment. But it should be noted that there is also a remarkable results obtained from the non-transplant setting with novel agent-based treatment, which later raised questions as to the role of upfront versus delayed ASCT [9].

Numerous rescue alternatives that incorporate distinctive combinations of medicines have been developed after the emergence of 2nd generation PIs and IMIDs, monoclonal antibodies (MAs), histone deacetylase inhibitors (HDIs), and, more as of late, check-point inhibitors (CPIs) and small molecules [17, 18]. These promising improvement requests a critical evaluation of treatment options to adequately top up the advantages of different induction, consolidation and maintenance approaches, and to set, a treatment ground so as to compare forthright ASCT, salvage ASCT and allotransplant in the era of novel agent [9].

Several drugs have shown promising activity against MM and are being used in clinical practice [19].

4.1 Induction therapy for ASCT-eligible patients

For patients with ASCT-eligible newly diagnosed MM, induction therapy with triple drugs should contain an IMiD, a PI, and a corticosteroid (Cs), usually lenalidomide-bortezomib-dexamethasone (RVd) [20]. The preferred induction therapy is combination of bortezomib with lenalidomide or thalidomide and dexamethasone (VRd or VTD), as well as the combination of daratumumab with VTD (DaraVTD) [21].

For patients presenting with renal impairment, cyclophophosphamide-bortezomib-dexamethasone is preferred, with the option to switch to RVd up on improvement of renal function. For patients intolerant to the triple therapy, double therapy can be used such as bortezomib-dexamethasone (Vd) and lenalidomide-dexamethasone (Rd), (**Figure 1**) [22].

Induction treatment can be administered for an extended period for up to 6–8 cycles [23]. A third drug can be added up on improvement of the patient started with two drugs. Recent data with carfilzomib-lenalidomide-dexamethasone (KRd) induction has shown much promise, and ongoing studies comparing the upfront KRd versus RVd have shown equivalent outcomes, if not improved [24].

Looking at the options of the novel triple (or quadruple) upfront Vs postpone for NDMM patients, it is widely advised that mobilization, stem cell harvest, conditioning and ASCT should be postponed due to the fear of immunosuppression in the upfront [25]. In patients receiving daratumumab and or lenalidomide-based induction, stem cell harvest without ASCT can be considered so as to achieve an adequate stem cell yield [8]. In this case, Granulocyte colony-stimulating factor (G-CSF) only mobilization with the potential addition of plerifaxor should be considered in order to avoid the immunosuppressive effect of high-dose cyclophosphamide. However, in cases of viral supra-infections like COVID-19, stem cell harvests and any transplant procedures should not be performed within at least 14, and preferably 21, days from the last contact (**Table 1**) [8].

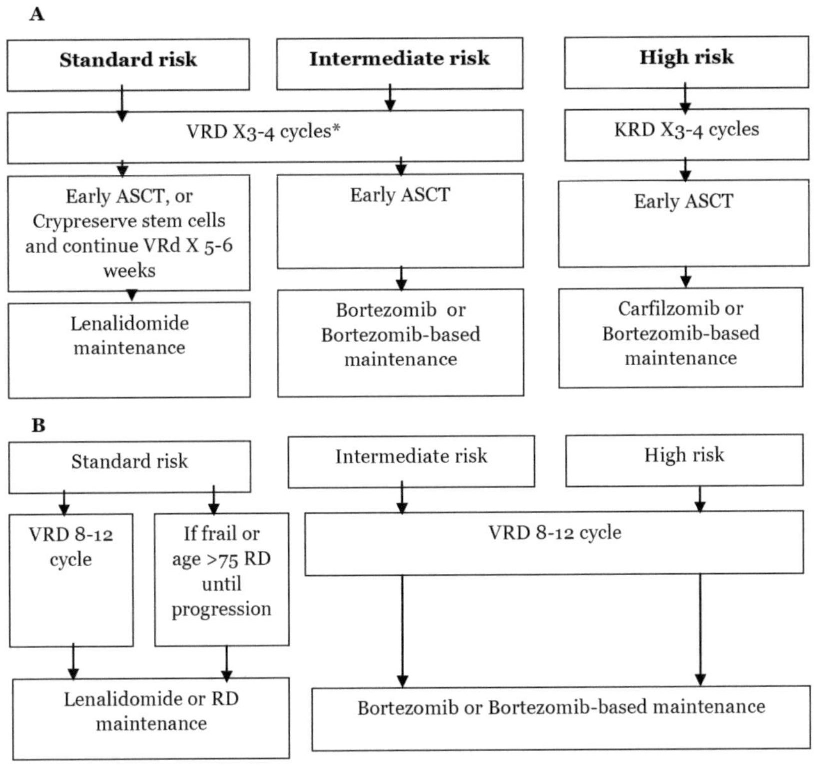

Figure 1.
Approach to the treatment of newly diagnosed multiple myeloma in transplant eligible A, and transplant ineligible B, patients. Abbreviations: ASCT, autologous stem cell transplantation; Dara-VRd, daratumumab, bortezomib, lenalidomide, dexamethasone; DRd, daratumumab, lenalidomide, dexamethasone; VRd, bortezomib, lenalidomide, dexamethasone [10].

The treatment schedule can be modified, for patients with sufficient response. Patients with high-risk disease features may receive ASCT after 6–8 induction cycles due to otherwise increased probability of progression [8]. Quadruple drugs trials are also offering good outcomes and will be available as alternative very soon [26].

4.2 Induction therapy for ASCT-ineligible patients

Patients who are fit or intermediate-fit to Rd. can be put on as a bridge therapy for 2–3 cycles in hospitals with peak prevalence of the current pandemic terror of the COVID-19. Otherwise, the approved VRd or daratumumab-based therapies (DaraRd or DaraVMP) can be administered. Dose of Dexamethasone should be lowered to 20 mg weekly, whereas de-escalation (or even interruption) can be made in patients responding well after the completion of 9 cycles of treatment [8]. Generally, RVd showed an excellent progression-free survival (PFS) and objective response rate (ORR). The triple therapy of daratumumab-lenalidomide-dexamethasone (DRd) showed much improved rates of partial response, better PFS, and tolerance compared to Rd. [27].

4.3 Treatment regimens

Wide ranges of regimens have been developed using a potentially effective combination of drugs that have proven efficacy in controlling disease progression and improving survival. The most commonly used drug combinations are listed in **Table 1**. The combinations are usually consists of IMIDs, Cs, PIs, and MAs targeting specific cell receptors like CD38, and are playing an important role in the management of MM [28].

Other active agents and approved for the treatment of MM include elotuzumab, a MA that is targeting the signaling lymphocytic activation molecule called SLAMF7 also known as CRACC, CS1, CD319*; panobinostat, a histone deacetylase inhibitor; selinexor, an inhibitor of exportin-1 called XPO1.; anthracyclines, doxorubicin and liposomal doxorubicin. However, elotuzumab, panobinostat, selinexor, and the anthracyclines do not have significant single-drug activity and hence should not be used individually; rather can be used to exert their therapeutic effect in combination with other active agents. Additionally, the anthracyclines are used infrequently in the treatment of MM because of the availability of other more active agents. In aggressive and refractory cases doxorubicin can be incorporated into some multi-agent combinations [19].

* CRACC: The CD2-like receptor-activating cytotoxic cell; CS1: subset 1.

4.4 Treatment algorithm

4.5 Consolidation therapy

The aim of consolidation is to increase the depth of response after induction, because achieving complete response or better is associated with improved survival (**Figure 1**) [16]. Consolidation may consist of ASCT (current standard of care for eligible patients) and/or single or multiple-drug agents after ASCT [29]. In ASCT-ineligible patients, consolidation may consist of single- or multiple-drug regimens [27].

Different types of stem-cell transplantations (SCT) has been used in MM including single ASCT, tandem ASCT, and, rarely, allogeneic stem-cell transplantation (alloSCT)) [30]. A three-arm trial that compared the outcome of RVd induction alone, single ASCT, and tandem ASCT, followed by all on lenalidomide maintenance therapy, unearthed that there was no differences on PFS and OS among all arm and concluded that the single ASCT followed by lenalidomide maintenance therapy has to be continued as the standard of care MM treatment [27].

For all eligible patients, after detail discussion on the outcomes of therapy, upfront ASCT can be used with four cycles of RVd followed by ASCT and four more cycles of RVd. Alternatively, eight cycles of RVd upfront, before ASCT can also be tried. Some patients prefer the latter option, to minimize treatment disruptions in case complications arise because of ASCT. If patients choose to defer upfront ASCT after being informed of the risks and benefits, then collection and storage of stem cells should be begun after four cycles of RVd [31].

4.6 Maintenance therapy

Maintenance therapy improves PFS and OS as compared to therapy cessation, indeed in high-risk patients [29, 32]. The survival benefit is present regardless of whether or not patients receive ASCT before maintenance. The use of maintenance does not seem to lead to decreased efficacy of therapy after first relapse and therefore is standard practice [29].

The IMWG reach on consensus that thalidomide maintenance therapy after ASCT improves the quality of response and increases the PFS as well as the OS significantly [33] though no improvement was seen in OS among elderly patients [33, 34].

Lenalidomide maintenance treatment after ASCT and after conventional melphalan, prednisone, and lenalidomide induction therapy showed a significant risk reduction of PFS as well as improvement in OS. Nevertheless, the role of thalidomide maintenance after induction therapy of melphalan, prednisone, and thalidomide is not yet well established [33].

Compared with conventional induction and thalidomide maintenance treatment a significantly increase in OS was seen with a bortezomib-based induction and bortezomib maintenance therapy after a single-agent bortezomib or in combination with thalidomide or prednisone maintenance therapy [35].

Appropriate therapeutic monitoring has to be taken so as to minimize drug associated toxicities during maintenance therapy. The risks and benefits should also be discussed with patients. Since there is no a single guiding principle reached as a consensus of standard care throughout all health care systems, clinical decisions for individual patients must be balanced with the potential benefits and risks specific management approach [36].

The standard agent for maintenance therapy of MM in U.S.A is lenalidomide, and maintenance therapy with lenalidomide is now favored following induction with or without ASCT because of prolonging response and improving PFS and OS. However, the risks with lenalidomide maintenance such as hematologic and solid secondary primary malignancies has to be given adequate focus [37].

Major trials of maintenance therapy for MM prescribed that all standard-risk patients have be managed with lenalidomide maintenance until improved. For high-risk patients, who are characterized as having either del (17p), t(4;14), or t(14;16), have be managed with dual maintenance comprising of lenalidomide and bortezomib each other week as long as safely endured. For patients with contraindications to bortezomib, ixazomib have to be considered once per weekly in lieu of bortezomib [38]. For very young and elderly patients systematic maintenance therapy is not recommended following induction because of the lack of sufficient data [39].

5. Prognostic factors

Cytogenetic abnormalities such as del(17p), t(14; 16), and t(14; 20) have important prognostic implications. Patients with del(17p), occurs in approximately 10% of newly diagnosed MM and in upwards of 80% in relapsed or refractory MM, are classified as high risk because of shortened OS and PFS [27]. Immunoglobulin heavy-chain translocations associated with the highest risk of poor outcomes include t(4;14) which is present in 5% and t(14;16) in 15% of newly diagnosed MM. Patients with both translocations are considered high risk and experience inferior survival [40].

The prognostic factors of MM is divided into four major parts as: 1) Risk Stratification, which includes Staging of MM, Plasma Cell Labeling index (PCLI), Cytogenetics and Gene Expression Profiling (GEP); 2) Monitoring of Response Tools, which includes Serum-Free Light Chain Assay, serum Heavy/Light Chain (HLC) Assay (Hevylite™), and Advanced Imaging Modalities; 3) Minimal Residual Disease (MRD) Monitoring Methods, which includes Circulating Plasma Cells, MRD Monitoring in General, and the Value of Depth of Response; and 4) Novel Prognostic Markers [41].

6. Management of relapsed and refractory cases

Treatment choice of a relapsed or refractory MM, depends on several parameters including age, the type of comorbidities, performance status, aggressiveness of relapse, efficacy and tolerance with the previously used medications, the number of prior drugs, the available remaining treatment options, the cytogenetic data at the time of relapse and the interval since the last therapy [27, 42].

Generally, During relapse a triple therapy is preferred over two drug treatment [43]. It should also be noted that, if patients relapse while receiving lenalidomide maintenance, carfilzomib-pomalidomide-dexamethasone and pomalidomide-bortezomib-dexamethasone are options in fit patients [44]. In transplant deferred cases, ASCT may be a good option [44].

For patients who were receiving bortezomib maintenance at the time of relapse or treatment failure, KRd may be used in fit patients. KRd demonstrated improved ORR, PFS, and OS in this population [45].

KRd and DRd may be considered for fit patients not receiving maintenance during relapse [46], and for frail patients or for those with indolent relapse ixazomib-lenalidomide-dexamethasone (IRd) or elotuzumab-lenalidomide-dexamethasone (ERd) may be considered [10, 46].

Pomalidomide-dexamethasone (Pd) is an option for patients with relapsed or refractory MM who have failed lenalidomide and bortezomib, and have received at least two prior therapies [47], the regimen improves PFS and OS in this population. The use of Pd in patients with relapsed or refractory MM who harbor del(17p) showed good prognostic factor [48].

Other combinations for relapsed or refractory MM include daratumumab-pomalidomide-dexamethasone, a PI with panobinostat, carfilzomib-cyclophosphamide-dexamethasone, and pomalidomide-cyclophosphamide-dexamethasone [27, 49].

For frail patients or for those with indolent relapse who relapsed during bortezomib maintenance, DRd, IRd, or ERd are effective [50]. Daratumumab-bortezomib-dexamethasone (DVd) or ixazomib-cyclophosphamide-dexamethasone are also options in frail patients [51].

Data comparing second ASCT to salvage therapy with novel PIs, IMiDs, or monoclonal antibodies not sufficient [17]. In addition, since lenalidomide maintenance is currently the standard of care after ASCT, the goal of considering a second transplantation should be closer to 36 months compared with 18 months on the basis of historical data [52]. If patients relapse after lenalidomide maintenance, considering a pomalidomide-based regimen, such as carfilzomib-pomalidomide-dexamethasone is recommended [27].

7. Supportive therapy

Supportive care is critical throughout the clinical course of patients with MM because they are particularly susceptible to infections. Diligence in identifying and initiating treatment at the earliest sign is advised [27].

All MM patients with newly diagnosed MM and with adequate renal function should be initiated with monthly bone-modulating therapy at diagnosis with either denosumab, zoledronic acid or pamidronate (high recommendation) [27].

Patients with clinical manifestation of MM but without objective evidence of lytic lesions using the conventional radiography can be managed with zoledronic acid (intermediate recommendations), though its advantages using the more advanced objective measurements like CT and MRI is not yet well established [53].

In patients without clinical manifestations of myeloma, the use of bisphonphonates is not generally advised (high evidence of toxicities) [8]. The continuous use of Zoledronic acid recommended as long as the cycles of treatments are on progress, but sufficient data are lacking supporting it after partial response to therapy is achieved [54, 55]. Denosumab doses can be administered at home if nursing facility is available or the patient should be trained for self-administration. Long-term discontinuation of denosumab treatment is associated with rebound effect and thus should be circumvented [8].

Sufficient data are available that prohibits the use of bortezomib-based regimens in patients with baseline clinical renal impairments. However, evidences are lacking supporting the discontinuation of therapy in patients who develop drug induced renal impairments [56, 57].

Severely anemic patients who do not respond to the conventional anemia management or deteriorating should be urgently switched to erythropoiesis stimulating agents (ESAs) in order to prevent the need for blood transfusions and frequent hospital visits. At present, the whole blood supplies has been extensively restricted due to the COVID-19 lockdown [8]. There are only few data advocating the use of ESAs in patients with persistent symptomatic anemia (hemoglobin <10 g/dL) where other causes of anemia have ruled out. Hence, ESAs should be discontinued after 6–8 weeks of therapy in patients' who fail to respond adequately to anemia treatment [58].

Immunization against influenza is recommended for specific infections caused by streptococcus pneumonia and hemophilus influenza, but sufficient data are lacking supporting the efficacy of the vaccination due to the fact that suboptimal immune responses are fairly seen after management [59].

If patients are receiving PIs & ASCT, the prophylactic use of antiviral agents such as acyclovir (or valacyclovir) are highly recommended [8, 60]. Acyclovir should be prescribed according to local protocols. Immunoglobulin administration may be given in an individualized basis, depending on the depth of suppression of polyclonal immunoglobulins and patient history of recurrent infections [34].

Antiviral prophylaxis has to be recommended in drugs associated with increased risk of herpes zoster reactivation such as Daratumumab and PIs. The prophylaxis is recommended for at least 3 months after exposure if no contraindications are observed [61].

Routine prophylaxis immunization should be considered with a series of pneumococcal conjugate vaccine 13 and pneumococcal polysaccharide vaccine, as well as annual influenza immunization [62]. Drugs such as IMiDs enhance the risk of venous thromboembolism, so preventive measures should be considered during active therapy [61], and the antithrombotic prophylaxis should be considered according to local or international guidelines. For countries with high incidence of COVID-19, low-molecular-weight heparin (LMWH) has to be preferred over aspirin as thromboprophylaxis in MM patients under IMiD administration, irrespective of their thrombotic risk [8, 63].

Patients with a history of neutropenias and/or recurrent infections should receive prophylactic G-CSF injections. Co-trimoxazole prophylaxis for Pneumocystis jirovecii for all patients and levofloxacin prophylaxis for the first three months of treatment for NDMM patients are also highly recommended [8, 55].

8. Follow-up and monitoring

Patients should be followed-up and monitored for complete blood counts (CBC), serum and urine electrophoresis with or without the use of serum-FLC determination, and also for serum calcium and creatinine measurements; at least in 2–3 months interval. In patients are complaining of bone pain, skeletal X-ray, MRI or CT scan should be carried out to detect and rule out new bone lesions [64].

9. Emerging role of targeted therapies, monoclonal antibodies, and cellular therapies

9.1 Venetoclax

Venetoclax is an orally bioavailable selective B-cell lymphoma 2 (Bcl-2) inhibitor. Bcl-2 and cyclin D1 are over expressed in MM patients with a translocation of (11;14), which is present in approximately 20% of patients with MM [65]. Venetoclax is an antiapoptotic protein and an emerging and effective treatment for relapsed or refractory MM [66, 67], and also being tried for treatment of chronic lymphocytic leukemia (CLL) cells [66] and non-Hodgkin lymphoma (NHL) [65]. Although response rates with venetoclax-dexamethasone are impressive in patients with t(11;14), PIs, which inhibit induced myeloid leukemia cell differentiation protein (Mcl-1), have synergistic activity when combined with venetoclax [27].

Currently the venetoclax is suspended by the Food and Drug Administration (FDA) because of a report obtained from the BELLINI trial, which stated an increased relative risk of death in the venetoclax group. As more recent data are being collected to have a better understanding of the safety concerns raised by the BELLINI trial [27, 68].

9.2 BRAF & BRAF/MEK inhibitors

BRAF is a proto-oncogene, that its protein product is a serine/threonine-protein kinase B-Raf that make conform the MAP kinase/ERKs signaling pathway, which works during cell division and differentiation [69]. In patients with MM, the incidence of BRAF V600E mutations is about 7–12% [70]. Trials evaluating BRAF and BRAF/MEK inhibitors in patients with MM harboring BRAF mutations are still undergoing [71].

9.3 Monoclonal antibodies (CAR T cells and BCMA)

Monoclonal antibodies represent an emerging class of agents in MM treatment [72]. Daratumumab-RVd versus RVd, are being evaluated for ASCT-eligible patients [27]. Isatuximab, a humanized immunoglobulin G1 monoclonal antibody, has distinct characteristics in contrast to other anti-CD38 monoclonal antibodies [72]. Isatuximab in combination with IMROZ, isatuximab-RVd in ASCT-ineligible patients with newly diagnosed MM are being studied [72]; and isatuximab-Kd (IKEMA) and isatuximab-Pd (ICARIA) have been tried in patients with relapsed or refractory MM [73].

B-cell maturation antigen (BCMA) is a significant target communicated on MM cells, with other targets counting GPR5CD, CD138, CD74, CD48, CD38, SLAMF7, and transmembrane activator and calcium modulator and cyclophilin ligand (CAML) interactor (TACI). Several strategies targeting BCMA include conjugated antibodies, cellular approaches, and bispecific T-cell engagers. Clinical trials evaluating BCMA-directed Chimeric antigen receptor redirected T cells (CAR-T cells) are furthest in development. Two notable BCMA CAR T-cell products are bb2121 and LCAR-B38M.69–71 Trials are evaluating CAR T cells in patients with relapsed or refractory MM to better understand their role in the MM treatment paradigm [74, 75].

Newly introduced therapies that uses CAR T cells and BCMA antibodies bid promises of adding agents to the antimyeloma armamentarium of neoadjuvant mechanisms of actions [49]. Enduring trials will permit for the integration of therapies with novel mechanisms of action, with the goal of inducing deeper responses as we endeavor towards the prospect of curative aspect of MM [27].

10. Conclusions

There is no cure for MM until today, however the recent advancements in management approaches provide hope for complete remission with improved survival. ASCT is currently considered the standard of care for fit newly diagnosed MM patients. Multiple combinations of PIs and IMIDs, salvaged with MAs, CTs, and other chemotherapeutic agents have been evaluated and available for both ASCT-eligibles as well as ineligible settings, while further studies are still running.

Acknowledgements

We are grateful for all researchers whom their invaluable works have been referenced to build up, construct and make in depth view of this book chapter.

Conflict of interest

The authors declare no conflict of interest.

Author details

Minyahil Alebachew Woldu*, Atalay Mulu Fentie and Tamrat Assefa Tadesse
Department of Pharmacology and Clinical Pharmacy, Addis Ababa University, Addis Ababa, Ethiopia

*Address all correspondence to: minyahil.alebachew@aau.edu.et

References

[1] Kumar SK, Callander NS, Alsina M, Atanackovic D, Biermann JS, Chandler JC, et al. Multiple myeloma, version 3.2017, NCCN clinical practice guidelines in oncology. Journal of the National Comprehensive Cancer Network. 2017;15(2):230-69. doi: https://doi.org/10.6004/jnccn.2017.0023.

[2] Kuehl WM, Bergsagel PL. Early genetic events provide the basis for a clinical classification of multiple myeloma. ASH Education Program Book. 2005;2005(1):346-52. doi: https://doi.org/10.1182/asheducation-2005.1.346.

[3] Willrich MA, Katzmann JA. Laboratory testing requirements for diagnosis and follow-up of multiple myeloma and related plasma cell dyscrasias. Clinical Chemistry and Laboratory Medicine (CCLM). 2016;54(6):907-19. doi: https://doi.org/10.1515/cclm-2015-0580.

[4] Harousseau J-L, Dreyling M. Multiple myeloma: ESMO Clinical Practice Guidelines for diagnosis, treatment and follow-up. Annals of Oncology. 2010;21:v155-v1v7. doi: 10.1093/annonc/mdq178.

[5] Moreau P, San Miguel J, Ludwig H, Schouten H, Mohty M, Dimopoulos M, et al. Multiple myeloma: ESMO Clinical Practice Guidelines for diagnosis, treatment and follow-up. Annals of Oncology. 2013;24:vi133-vi7. doi: 10.1093/annonc/mdt297.

[6] Rajkumar SV. Multiple myeloma: 2016 update on diagnosis, risk-stratification, and management. American journal of hematology. 2016;91(7):719-734. doi: 10.1002/ajh.24402.

[7] Terpos E, Kleber M, Engelhardt M, Zweegman S, Gay F, Kastritis E, et al. European Myeloma Network guidelines for the management of multiple myeloma-related complications. Haematologica. 2015;100(10):1254-1266. doi: 10.3324/haematol.2014.117176.

[8] Terpos E, Engelhardt M, Cook G, Gay F, Mateos M-V, Ntanasis-Stathopoulos I, et al. Management of patients with multiple myeloma in the era of COVID-19 pandemic: a consensus paper from the European Myeloma Network (EMN). Leukemia. 2020;34(8):2000-11. doi: https://doi.org/10.1038/s41375-020-0876-z.

[9] Gay F, Engelhardt M, Terpos E, Wäsch R, Giaccone L, Auner HW, et al. From transplant to novel cellular therapies in multiple myeloma: European Myeloma Network guidelines and future perspectives. Haematologica. 2018;103(2):197. doi: 10.3324/haematol.2017.174573.

[10] Rajkumar SV. Multiple myeloma: 2020 update on diagnosis, risk-stratification and management. American journal of hematology. 2020;95(5):548-67. doi: https://doi.org/10.1002/ajh.25791.

[11] San-Miguel JF, Paiva B, Gutiérrez NC. New tools for diagnosis and monitoring of multiple myeloma. Am Soc Clin Oncol Educ Book. 2013;10:12-15.

[12] Fowler NH, Staudt LM, Bradner J. Hot Pathways for Targeted Therapy of B-Cell Malignancies. American Society of Clinical Oncology Educational Book. 2013.

[13] Rajkumar SV, Dimopoulos MA, Palumbo A, Blade J, Merlini G, Mateos M-V, et al. International Myeloma Working Group updated criteria for the diagnosis of multiple myeloma. The lancet oncology. 2014;15(12):e538-e48.

doi: https://doi.org/10.1016/S1470-2045(14)70442-5.

[14] Lentzsch S, O'Sullivan A, Kennedy RC, Abbas M, Dai L, Pregja SL, et al. Combination of bendamustine, lenalidomide, and dexamethasone (BLD) in patients with relapsed or refractory multiple myeloma is feasible and highly effective: results of phase 1/2 open-label, dose escalation study. Blood, The Journal of the American Society of Hematology. 2012;119(20):4608-13. doi: https://doi.org/10.1182/blood-2011-12-395715.

[15] Davidson HC. Serotonin is a survival factor for human multiple myeloma cells. Drexel University College of Medicine; 2004.

[16] Durie BG. Role of new treatment approaches in defining treatment goals in multiple myeloma–the ultimate goal is extended survival. Cancer treatment reviews. 2010;36:S18-S23. doi: https://doi.org/10.1016/S0305-7372(10)70008-6.

[17] Chim C, Kumar S, Orlowski R, Cook G, Richardson P, Gertz M, et al. Management of relapsed and refractory multiple myeloma: novel agents, antibodies, immunotherapies and beyond. Leukemia. 2018;32(2):252-262.

[18] Cetani G, Boccadoro M, Oliva S. A look at treatment strategies for relapsed multiple myeloma. Expert review of anticancer therapy. 2018;18(8):735-50. doi: https://doi.org/10.1080/14737140.2018.1477594.

[19] Rajkumar SV, Kumar S. Multiple myeloma current treatment algorithms. Blood cancer journal. 2020;10(9):1-10.

[20] Bagal B, Bonda A. Induction therapy in newly diagnosed multiple myeloma: Current research scenario and questions for the future. Cancer Research, Statistics, and Treatment. 2019;2(1):76. doi: 10.4103/CRST.CRST_42_19.

[21] Paul B, Lipe B, Ocio EM, Usmani SZ. Induction therapy for newly diagnosed multiple myeloma. American Society of Clinical Oncology Educational Book. 2019;39:e176-ee86. doi: 10.1200/EDBK_238527.

[22] Chari A, Parikh K, Ni Q, Abouzaid S. Treatment patterns and clinical and economic outcomes in patients with newly diagnosed multiple myeloma treated with lenalidomide- and/or bortezomib-containing regimens without stem cell transplant in a real-world setting. Clinical Lymphoma Myeloma and Leukemia. 2019;19(10):645-55. doi: https://doi.org/10.1016/j.clml.2019.06.007.

[23] Moreau P, Pylypenko H, Grosicki S, Karamanesht I, Leleu X, Grishunina M, et al. Subcutaneous versus intravenous administration of bortezomib in patients with relapsed multiple myeloma: a randomised, phase 3, non-inferiority study. The lancet oncology. 2011;12(5):431-40. doi: https://doi.org/10.1016/S1470-2045(11)70081-X.

[24] Dimopoulos MA, Jakubowiak AJ, McCarthy PL, Orlowski RZ, Attal M, Bladé J, et al. Developments in continuous therapy and maintenance treatment approaches for patients with newly diagnosed multiple myeloma. Blood cancer journal. 2020;10(2):1-19. doi: https://doi.org/10.1038/s41408-020-0273-x.

[25] Goldschmidt H, Ashcroft J, Szabo Z, Garderet L. Navigating the treatment landscape in multiple myeloma: which combinations to use and when? Annals of hematology. 2019;98(1):1-18. doi: https://doi.org/10.1007/s00277-018-3546-8.

[26] Cohen YC, Zada M, Gatt ME, Lavi N, Ganzel C, Wang S-Y, et al. Kydar

multicenter trial of quadruple regimen for induction resistant myeloma combined with translational single-cell analysis identifies potential drivers of advanced resistance, including novel immune checkpoints. American Society of Hematology Washington, DC; 2019.

[27] Branagan A, Lei M, Lou U, Raje N. Current Treatment Strategies for Multiple Myeloma. JCO Oncology Practice. 2020;16(1):5-14. doi: 10.1200/jop.19.00244.

[28] Leclercq R, Courvalin P. Resistance to glycopeptides in enterococci. Clinical Infectious Diseases. 1997;24(4): 545-554.

[29] Palumbo A, Cavallo F, Gay F, Di Raimondo F, Ben Yehuda D, Petrucci MT, et al. Autologous transplantation and maintenance therapy in multiple myeloma. New England Journal of Medicine. 2014;371(10):895-905.

[30] Armand P, Kim HT, Logan BR, Wang Z, Alyea EP, Kalaycio ME, et al. Validation and refinement of the Disease Risk Index for allogeneic stem cell transplantation. Blood. 2014;123(23):3664-71. doi: https://doi.org/10.1182/blood-2014-01-552984.

[31] Cavo M, Rajkumar SV, Palumbo A, Moreau P, Orlowski R, Bladé J, et al. International Myeloma Working Group consensus approach to the treatment of multiple myeloma patients who are candidates for autologous stem cell transplantation. Blood. 2011;117(23): 6063-6073.

[32] Sivaraj D, Green MM, Li Z, Sung AD, Sarantopoulos S, Kang Y, et al. Outcomes of maintenance therapy with bortezomib after autologous stem cell transplantation for patients with multiple myeloma. Biology of Blood and Marrow Transplantation. 2017; 23(2):262-8. doi: https://doi.org/10.1016/j.bbmt.2016.11.010.

[33] Ludwig H, Durie BG, McCarthy P, Palumbo A, San Miguel J, Barlogie B, et al. IMWG consensus on maintenance therapy in multiple myeloma. Blood. 2012;119(13):3003-15. doi: ttps://doi.org/10.1182/blood-2011-11-374249.

[34] Engelhardt M, Terpos E, Kleber M, Gay F, Wäsch R, Morgan G, et al. European Myeloma Network recommendations on the evaluation and treatment of newly diagnosed patients with multiple myeloma. haematologica. 2014;99(2):232. doi: doi: 10.3324/haematol.2013.099358.

[35] Kapoor P, Ramakrishnan V, Rajkumar SV. Bortezomib combination therapy in multiple myeloma. Seminars in hematology: Elsevier; 2012. p. 228-242.

[36] Chou R, Fanciullo GJ, Fine PG, Adler JA, Ballantyne JC, Davies P, et al. Clinical guidelines for the use of chronic opioid therapy in chronic noncancer pain. The Journal of Pain. 2009;10(2): 113-30. e22. doi: https://doi.org/10.1016/j.jpain.2008.10.008.

[37] Dhakal B, Szabo A, Chhabra S, Hamadani M, D'Souza A, Usmani SZ, et al. Autologous transplantation for newly diagnosed multiple myeloma in the era of novel agent induction: a systematic review and meta-analysis. JAMA oncology. 2018;4(3):343-350. doi: 10.1001/jamaoncol.2017.4600.

[38] Sonneveld P, Avet-Loiseau H, Lonial S, Usmani S, Siegel D, Anderson KC, et al. Treatment of multiple myeloma with high-risk cytogenetics: a consensus of the International Myeloma Working Group. Blood. 2016;127(24):2955-62. doi: https://doi.org/10.1182/blood-2016-01-631200.

[39] Wang Y, Yang F, Shen Y, Zhang W, Wang J, Chang VT, et al. Maintenance therapy with immunomodulatory drugs in multiple myeloma: a meta-analysis

and systematic review. Journal of the National Cancer Institute. 2016;108(3):djv342. doi: https://doi.org/10.1093/jnci/djv342.

[40] Warsame R, Kumar SK, Gertz M, Lacy M, Buadi F, Hayman S, et al. Abnormal FISH in patients with immunoglobulin light chain amyloidosis is a risk factor for cardiac involvement and for death. Blood cancer journal. 2015;5(5):e310-e. doi: https://doi.org/10.1038/bcj.2015.34.

[41] Hanbali A, Hassanein M, Rasheed W, Aljurf M, Alsharif F. The evolution of prognostic factors in multiple myeloma. Advances in hematology. 2017;2017. doi: https://doi.org/10.1155/2017/4812637.

[42] Moreau P. How I treat myeloma with new agents. Blood. 2017;130(13):1507-13. doi: https://doi.org/10.1182/blood-2017-05-743203.

[43] Nijhof IS, van de Donk NW, Zweegman S, Lokhorst HM. Current and new therapeutic strategies for relapsed and refractory multiple myeloma: an update. Drugs. 2018;78(1):19-37.

[44] Chung C. Role of immunotherapy in targeting the bone marrow microenvironment in multiple myeloma: an evolving therapeutic strategy. Pharmacotherapy: The Journal of Human Pharmacology and Drug Therapy. 2017;37(1):129-143.

[45] Raza S, Safyan RA, Rosenbaum E, Bowman AS, Lentzsch S. Optimizing current and emerging therapies in multiple myeloma: a guide for the hematologist. Therapeutic advances in hematology. 2017;8(2):55-70.

[46] Rajkumar SV. Multiple myeloma: 2018 update on diagnosis, risk-stratification, and management. American journal of hematology. 2018;93(8):1091-1110.

[47] Richardson PG, Siegel DS, Vij R, Hofmeister CC, Baz R, Jagannath S, et al. Pomalidomide alone or in combination with low-dose dexamethasone in relapsed and refractory multiple myeloma: a randomized phase 2 study. Blood, The Journal of the American Society of Hematology. 2014;123(12):1826-1832.

[48] Ziogas DC, Dimopoulos MA, Kastritis E. Prognostic factors for multiple myeloma in the era of novel therapies. Expert review of hematology. 2018;11(11):863-879.

[49] Lei M, Kim EB, Branagan A, Lou U, Zemel M, Raje N. Current management and emerging treatment strategies for multiple myeloma. Rinsho Ketsueki. 2019;60(9):1243-1256.

[50] Dingli D, Ailawadhi S, Bergsagel PL, Buadi FK, Dispenzieri A, Fonseca R, et al. Therapy for relapsed multiple myeloma: guidelines from the Mayo stratification for myeloma and risk-adapted therapy. Mayo Clinic Proceedings: Elsevier; 2017. p. 578-598.

[51] Mukherjee D, Mukherjee KK. A Review on Therapeutic strategies of Relapsed and Refractory Multiple Myeloma. 2021.

[52] Moreau P, Zamagni E, Mateos M-V. Treatment of patients with multiple myeloma progressing on frontline-therapy with lenalidomide. Blood cancer journal. 2019;9(4):1-8.

[53] Coleman R, Brown J, Terpos E, Lipton A, Smith MR, Cook R, et al. Bone markers and their prognostic value in metastatic bone disease: clinical evidence and future directions. Cancer treatment reviews. 2008;34(7):629-639.

[54] Terpos E, Kleber M, Engelhardt M, Zweegman S, Gay F, Kastritis E, et al. European Myeloma Network guidelines for the management of multiple

myeloma-related complications. haematologica. 2015;100(10):1254.

[55] Morgan GJ, Davies FE, Gregory WM, Cocks K, Bell SE, Szubert AJ, et al. First-line treatment with zoledronic acid as compared with clodronic acid in multiple myeloma (MRC Myeloma IX): a randomised controlled trial. The Lancet. 2010;376(9757):1989-1999.

[56] Beirão I, Costa PP. Erythropoietin in Familial Amyloidosis ATTR V30M. Erythropoietic Stimulating Agents. 2013;1:1144.

[57] Talmadge JE. Natural product derived immune-regulatory agents. International immunopharmacology. 2016;37:5-15.

[58] Beguin Y, Dujardin C, Piron M, Vanstraelen G. Treatment of anaemia with erythropoietin. ESH Scientific Updates Disorders of Iron Homeostasis, Erythrocytes and erythropoiesis. 2006:180-209.

[59] Westerink MJ, Schroeder Jr HW, Nahm MH. Immune responses to pneumococcal vaccines in children and adults: rationale for age-specific vaccination. Aging and disease. 2012;3(1):51.

[60] Beksaç M. European myeloma network guidelines for the management of multiple myeloma-related complications. 2015. doi: https://doi.org/10.3324/haematol.2014.117176.

[61] Nahi H, Chrobok M, Gran C, Lund J, Gruber A, Gahrton G, et al. Infectious complications and NK cell depletion following daratumumab treatment of multiple myeloma. PloS one. 2019;14(2):e0211927. doi: https://doi.org/10.1371/journal.pone.0211927.

[62] Ludwig H, Boccadoro M, Moreau P, San-Miguel J, Cavo M, Pawlyn C, et al. Recommendations for vaccination in multiple myeloma: a consensus of the European Myeloma Network. Leukemia. 2020:1-14.

[63] Palumbo A, Sezer O, Kyle R, Miguel J, Orlowski R, Moreau P, et al. International Myeloma Working Group guidelines for the management of multiple myeloma patients ineligible for standard high-dose chemotherapy with autologous stem cell transplantation. Leukemia. 2009;23(10):1716-30. doi: https://doi.org/10.1038/leu.2009.122.

[64] Moreau P, San Miguel J, Sonneveld P, Mateos M-V, Zamagni E, Avet-Loiseau H, et al. Multiple myeloma: ESMO Clinical Practice Guidelines for diagnosis, treatment and follow-up. Annals of Oncology. 2017;28:iv52-iv61. doi: 10.1200/JCO.2016.70.4320.

[65] Davids MS, Roberts AW, Seymour JF, Pagel JM, Kahl BS, Wierda WG, et al. Phase I first-in-human study of venetoclax in patients with relapsed or refractory non-Hodgkin lymphoma. Journal of Clinical Oncology. 2017;35(8):826. doi: 10.1200/JCO.2016.70.4320.

[66] Seymour JF, Kipps TJ, Eichhorst B, Hillmen P, D'Rozario J, Assouline S, et al. Venetoclax–rituximab in relapsed or refractory chronic lymphocytic leukemia. New England Journal of Medicine. 2018;378(12):1107-1120. doi: 10.1056/NEJMoa1713976.

[67] Wudhikarn K, Wills B, Lesokhin AM. Monoclonal antibodies in multiple myeloma: Current and emerging targets and mechanisms of action. Best Practice & Research Clinical Haematology. 2020;33(1):101143. doi: https://doi.org/10.1016/j.beha.2020.101143.

[68] Saturni S, Bellini F, Braido F, Paggiaro P, Sanduzzi A, Scichilone N, et al. Randomized controlled trials and real life studies. Approaches and

methodologies: a clinical point of view. Pulmonary pharmacology & therapeutics. 2014;27(2):129-38. doi: https://doi.org/10.1016/j.pupt.2014.01.005.

[69] Domingo E, Schwartz Jr S. BRAF (v-raf murine sarcoma viral oncogene homolog B1. Atlas of Genetics and Cytogenetics in Oncology and Haematology. 2004.

[70] Lee S-T, Kim SW, Ki C-S, Jang J-H, Shin JH, Oh YL, et al. Clinical implication of highly sensitive detection of the BRAF V600E mutation in fine-needle aspirations of thyroid nodules: a comparative analysis of three molecular assays in 4585 consecutive cases in a BRAF V600E mutation-prevalent area. The Journal of Clinical Endocrinology & Metabolism. 2012;97(7):2299-306. doi: https://doi.org/10.1210/jc.2011-3135.

[71] Baik CS, Myall NJ, Wakelee HA. Targeting BRAF-mutant non-small cell lung cancer: From molecular profiling to rationally designed therapy. The oncologist. 2017;22(7):786. doi: 10.1634/theoncologist.2016-0458.

[72] van de Donk NW, Janmaat ML, Mutis T, Lammerts van Bueren JJ, Ahmadi T, Sasser AK, et al. Monoclonal antibodies targeting CD 38 in hematological malignancies and beyond. Immunological reviews. 2016;270(1):95-112. doi: https://doi.org/10.1111/imr.12389.

[73] Cavo M. Facing lenalidomide-refractory myeloma. Blood, The Journal of the American Society of Hematology. 2019;134(2):99-101. doi: https://doi.org/10.1182/blood-2019-04-901157.

[74] Shah N, Chari A, Scott E, Mezzi K, Usmani SZ. B-cell maturation antigen (BCMA) in multiple myeloma: rationale for targeting and current therapeutic approaches. Leukemia. 2020;34(4):985-1005. doi: https://doi.org/10.1038/s41375-020-0734-z.

[75] Huehls AM, Coupet TA, Sentman CL. Bispecific T-cell engagers for cancer immunotherapy. Immunology and cell biology. 2015;93(3):290-6. doi: https://doi.org/10.1038/icb.2014.93.

Chapter 4

Antibody Therapies for Multiple Myeloma

Nikolaos Kanellias, Maria Gavriatopoulou and Evangelos Terpos

Abstract

Multiple Myeloma (MM) is characterized by the abberant proliferation and expansion of plasma cells in the Bone marrow. Despite the broad use of proteasome inhibitors and IMiDs, Multiple Myeloma remains an incurable disease. The introduction of Monoclonal antibodies, along with bi-specific antibodies and check point inhibitors, has significantly enhanced the armamentarium of available therapeutic options in the relapsed setting. The incorporation of the abovementioned novel agents in triplet or quadruplet therapeutic regimens has led to significant prolongation of overall survival (OS) and progression free survival (PFS), without adding significant toxicity. Anti-CD38 monoclonal antibodies has become the cornerstone of antimyeloma therapy in both the newly diagnosed and relapsed setting.

Keywords: Monoclonal Antibodies, Antibody Drug Conjugates, Daratumumab, Belantamab Mafodotin

1. Introduction

Multiple Myeloma is characterized by the upregulation and expansion of plasma cells malignant clones in the bone marrow [1]. The introduction of novel agents such as immunomodulatory drugs (IMiDs) and proteasome inhibitors (PIs) has led to significant improvement of disease prognosis and survival. However, the disease remains incurable, and all patients will relapse. Patients who are refractory to both Imids and PIs have poor survival outcomes, with a median overall survival of 9–13 months [2, 3]. The identification of novel therapeutic approaches for this group of patients represents an unmet medical need. In addition to that, patients with advanced disease characteristics and high-risk cytogenetics have a poor prognosis [4, 5]. Immune dysregulation represents a hallmark of MM pathophysiology. A better understanding of mechanisms that govern immune impairment in MM, has led to the development of several immunotherapeutic agents such as monoclonal antibodies, bispecific antibodies (BiTEs), and chimeric antigen receptor (CAR) T-cells.

2. Monoclonal antibodies

2.1 Daratumumab

2.1.1 Daratumumab mechanism of action

Daratumumab (Dara) is the first in class humanized IgG1-κ monoclonal antibody targeting CD38 through binding to a unique epitope which includes amino acids 233–246 and 267–280 [6]. Following binding to CD38, Dara exerts its action through canonical (classical) and noncanonical mechanisms [7]. Canonical mechanisms are immune-mediated, dependent on Dara binding to CD38 on the tumor cell, and include complement-mediated cytotoxicity (CDC), antibody-dependent cell-mediated cytotoxicity (ADCC), antibody-dependent cell-mediated phagocytosis (ADCP), direct cytotoxicity upon secondary cross-linking, and inhibition of CD38 enzymatic activity. Canonical mechanisms could be either Fcgamma receptor (FcgR) dependent or independent [6, 8, 9]. Whilst the canonical mechanisms explain the activity of Dara against CD38+ cells, noncanonical mechanisms are independent of Dara binding to CD38 and based on modulation of immune cells [10]. Dara targets three main categories of immunosuppressor cells that express CD38. These categories are Regulatory B cells (Bregs), which promote tumor growth and immune escape, a subset of regulatory T cells (Tregs), and Myeloid-derived suppressor cells (MDSC). After Dara binding to the CD38 in the surface of the above-mentioned cells causes depletion of their population [11]. Following the depletion of regulatory cells, there is a significant increase in the populations of CD4+ and CD8+ effector T-cells [12–15]. Effector T-cells have increased levels of granzyme-B, which results in enhanced killing capacity [12, 16].

2.1.2 Daratumumab combinations in the newly diagnosed setting

2.1.2.1 Transplant-ineligible patients

The combination of bortezomib melphalan and prednisone (VMP) is considered a standard of care regimen for patients who are not candidates for transplant. ALCYONE (NCT02195479) is a phase 3 trial in which patients with NDMM were randomized to receive bortezomib melphalan and prednisone either alone or in combination with Dara. The primary endpoint was PFS. The comparison of PFS rates at 16.5 and 40.08 months showed a sustained superiority of Dara-VMP versus VMP groups. At 16.5 and 40.08 months, PFS rates for Dara VMP and VMP groups were 71.6% (95% [CI], 65.5 to 76.8) vs. 50.2% (95% CI, 43.2 to 56.7) and 36.4 vs. 19.3 months respectively [17, 18]. At the time point of 40.08 months, the median PFS2 was not reached versus 42.3 months for the Dara-VMP and the VMP arm, respectively 32376237. The combination of Dara-VMP also demonstrated a significant reduction in the risk of death by 40% in comparison with VMP (HR 0.60 95% CI 0.46–0.80; p = 0·0003) [19]. At the time point of 42 months, the estimated overall survival rate in Dara-VMP and VMP groups was 75% vs. 62% (median not reached in either group HR: 0.60; 95% CI: 0.46 to 0.80; P = 0.0003) respectively [17, 18, 20]. The proportion of patients achieving MRD negativity was better in the Dara-VMP group (28% versus 7%) 32376237 After a median follow-up of 40.1 months, Dara-VMP increased the ORR (90.9% vs. 73.9%) and the rates of ≥VGPR (73% vs. 50%), ≥CR (46% vs. 25%), MRD-negativity (28% vs. 7%; all P < 0.0001), and ≥ CR with MRD-negativity (27% vs. 7%) vs. VMP. Time to subsequent therapy, OS, and PFS was prolonged for patients with deeper responses in both groups Alcyone 2020.

MAIA trial (NCT02252172) is a phase 3 trial in which the addition of Dara to Rd. was compared to Rd. alone. Seven hundred thirty-seven patients who were ineligible for transplant were recruited. Patients were randomly assigned to receive Rd. with or without Dara in 28-day cycles until disease progression or unacceptable toxicity. The primary end-point was progression-free survival [21]. Results from the primary analysis (median follow-up 28 months) showed that the addition of Dara to Rd. improved PFS and MRD-negativity rates. After a longer follow up period (36.4 months), patients in the DRd arm maintained deeper and durable response along with PFS benefit [22]. After a median follow-up of 47.9 months, patients in the DRd arm had better PFS in comparison with the control group (median, not reached [NR] vs. 34 mo; HR, 0.54; 95% CI, 0.43–0.67; P < 0.0001). Median PFS2 was not reached for DRd vs. 51 months in the Rd. arm. (HR, 0.65; 95% CI, 0.52–0.83; P = 0.0005). The addition of Dara to Rd. resulted in deeper responses with higher rates of CR or better and VGPR or better. The median duration of response was not reached for responders in the DRd arm vs. 44 months in the Rd. arm [23].

2.1.2.2 Transplant-eligible patients

The combination of Dara Bortezomib, cyclophosphamide, and dexamethasone (Dara-VCD) resulted in ORR and VGPR or better rates of 81% and 56%, respectively, in NDMM patients enrolled in the LYRA (NCT02951819) study 30828799. After 6–8 cycles of Dara-VCD induction, eligible patients underwent ASCT. All patients received Dara maintenance. The administration of Dara as maintenance therapy improved the depth of response and was associated with prolongation of both PFS and OS [24].

GRIFFIN (NCT02874742) is a phase 2 trial evaluating the addition of Dara to the induction regimen Bortezomib Lenalidomide and Dexamethasone (VRD) in NDMM transplant eligible patients. Patients were randomized to receive Dara-VRD or VRD as induction regimen, ASCT, two cycles of Dara-VRD or VRD consolidation, and Revlimid alone or in combination with Dara as maintenance for 24 cycles. The primary endpoint was the rate of s CR post-consolidation. Regarding the randomized phase of the trial, results indicated that the combination of Dara-VRD was safe and potent. Regarding the primary endpoint results favored the quadruplet regimen (D-VRD)) 42 patients (42.4%) in the D-VRD and 31 patients (32.0%) in the VRD group achieved sCR by the end of consolidation (odds ratio, 1.57; 95% [CI], 0.87–2.82 1-sided P = .068) Response improved over time. After a median follow up of 22.1 months, the sCR (62.6% vs. 45.4%; P = .0177) and MRD negativity (51.0% vs. 20.4%; P < .0001, threshold 10^{-5}) improved in the D-VRD arm in the intent to treat population [25]. In the final analysis of the safety run-in cohort, at the end of consolidation, 9 (56.3%) patients achieved sCR, and 8 (50.0%) were MRD negative (10–5 threshold). After maintenance, 15 (93.8%) patients achieved sCR, and 13 (81.3%) were MRD (10^{-5}) negative. Estimated 36-month overall and progression-free survival rates were 93.8% and 78.1%, respectively. Results showed that the addition of Dara to R AND VRD resulted in durable responses and sustained MRD negativity. The depth of response improved over time [26].

CASSIOPEIA (NCT02541383) is an ongoing phase III clinical trial in newly diagnosed transplant eligible MM patients divided into two parts. Patients were randomized to receive four pre-transplant induction and two post-transplant consolidation cycles of VTd with (VTd group) or without daratumumab (D-VTd group). The primary endpoint of part 1 was the Scr rate assessed 100 days after transplantation. Part 2 (maintenance) is ongoing. After completion of induction and consolidation, the sCR rate in the D-VTd group was 28.9% vs. 20.3% in the VTd group (odds ratio 1.60, 95%CI 1.21–2.12, p = 0.0010). Additionally, the D-VTd group had significantly prolonged PFS in comparison with VTd (HR: 0.47; 95%CI: 0.33–0.67, p < 0.0001) [27].

MASTER (NCT03224507) is an ongoing phase II clinical trial. Newly diagnosed transplant eligible MM patients received four cycles of Dara-Carfilzomib Dexamethasone (Dara-KRD) induction, followed by autologous stem cell transplantation (ASCT) and consolidation with Dara-KRD based on the MRD status. The MRD assessment method was next-generation sequencing (NGS), and the threshold was 10^{-5}. Evaluation of MRD status was performed at specific time points. At the end of the induction, post ASCT and post cycles 4 and 8 of consolidation. Patients with two consecutive negative MRD results stopped treatment. Patients who concluded treatment underwent imaging. The administration of Dara-KRD resulted in rapid and durable responses. More than 90% of patients achieved VGPR or better response by the end of induction. The MRD negative rates at the end of induction at ASCT and at best response were 34%, 70%, and 80% (threshold 10^{-5}) and 28%, 45%, and 65% (threshold 10^{-6}), respectively. Until today 11 patients have concluded treatment after achieving MRD negativity without evidence of relapse. The trial is ongoing, and long term follow up results are awaited [28].

PERSEUS (NCT03710603) is a randomized, phase 3 study comparing DARA-VRd vs. VRd in transplant eligible NDMM patients, which has recently concluded its enrollment of patients. PFS is the primary endpoint, while key secondary endpoints include, ORR, MRD-negative rate and OS.

2.1.3 Daratumumab combinations in the R/R setting

POLLUX (NCT02076009) is a phase III clinical trial that compared the combination of Lenalidomide Dexamethasone with or without daratumumab in MM patients who had received at least one prior line of treatment and were not refractory to Lenalidomide [15]. The addition of Dara significantly improved PFS at 12 (83.2%, 95% CI, 78.3 to 87.2 vs. 60.1%, 95% CI, 54.0 to 65.7), 25,4 (median not reached vs. 17.5 months; HR 0.41; 95% CI,0.31–0.53; P < 0.0001) and 44,3 (median 44.5 vs. 17.5 months; HR, 0.44; 95% CI, 0.35–0.55; P < 0.0001) months follow up in comparison with the control group [15, 29, 30]. The overall response rate was significantly better in the DRd group (92.9% vs. 76.4%, P < 0.001) 30237262. Post hoc analyses revealed that Dara improved PFS independently of the prior lines of treatment and high-risk cytogenetics [29]. At 25.4 months, the assessment of MRD status (threshold 10^{-5}) revealed deeper responses in the DRd arm (26.2% vs. 6.4% P < 0.0001) [29].

CASTOR study (NCT02136134) compared the combination of Dara Vd (Dvd) versus Vd in 498 patients who had received at least one prior line of therapy (median of 2, range, 1–10; 10% three or more) and were not Bortezomib refractory. The study met its primary endpoint with a significant prolongation of PFS in the Dvd group after 7.4 months follow up (not reached in the Dvd versus 7.2 months in the Vd group), along with a significant reduction (61%) regarding the risk of disease progression or death (HR: 0.39; 95% CI, 0.28–0.53; p < 0.001). ORR was 82.9% in the Dvd vs. 63.2% in the Vd group, P < 0.001 [31]. Updated results of this trial after 40 months, reinforce the tolerability and effectiveness of Dvd. PFS was improved in all subgroups (16.7 vs. 7.1 months, [HR], 0.31; 95% [CI], 0.25–0.40; P < .0001). 32482541. The addition of Dara to Vd manage to overcome the impact of high-risk cytogenetic abnormalities (12.6 vs. 6.2 months; HR, 0.41; 95% CI, 0.21–0.83; P = 0.0106) 32819447 Patients in the Dvd group had 2.5 fold higher MRD negativity rate (10–5 threshold) [31]. Based on the results of CASTOR trial FDA and EMA approved in 2016 Dvd for RRMM patients who had received at least one prior line of treatment.

In a phase 1b study (MMY1001), the addition of Dara to Pomalidomide and Dexamethasone was tested. The study included 103 patients with a median age of 64 years and a median of four prior lines of therapy. Notably, 89% were refractory to Lenalidomide, 71% to Bortezomib, and 30% to Carfilzomib. The median OS and PFS were 17,5 and 8,8 months, respectively. The ORR was 60%. The combination of Dara Pom Dex was clearly safe and effective in this group of heavily pretreated patients [32]. Based on these results, FDA approved this triple combination for patients who had received at least two prior lines, including both a PI and Lenalidomide [32].

APOLLO trial (NCT03180736) explored the addition of Dara to Pomalidomide and dexamethasone (Pd) in 304 patients with RRMM who had received ≥one prior line of therapy, including a PI and Lenalidomide. PFS was the primary endpoint. Patients received Pomalidomide 4 mg d1–21, dexamethasone 40 mg (20 mg for patients ≥75 years of age) on 28 days cycles. Patients initially received Daratumumab iv 16 mg/kg. After protocol amendment, patients continued with Dara sc 1800 mg. Administration of Dara every week for cycles one and two, every two weeks for cycles 3–6, and every month thereafter. Prior Pomalidomide or anti-CD-38 administration was not permitted. The patient's median age was 67 (35–90) years, 35% had high-risk cytogenetics, and 63% were refractory to both Len and PI. The study met its primary endpoint. The addition of Dara to Pd led to a significant prolongation of PFS (12.4 months) versus 6.9 months in the Pd arm (HR 0.63 (95% CI, 0.47–0.85; P = 0.0018), which represents a 37% reduction in the risk of death or progression. Data regarding OS are immature, and longer follow-up is warranted. No new safety signals have emerged. Additionally, the sc formulation of Dara shortens the duration of administration. These data suggest that the D-Pd combination is safe, effective, and convenient in the RR setting [33].

CANDOR (NCT03158688) is another phase 3 trial exploring the addition of Dara to Carfilzomib and dexamethasone (Kd). Four hundred sixty-six patients were randomized to receive Dara Carfilzomib dexamethasone (DKd) vs. Kd. All patients received iv Dara at 16 mg/kg, every week for the first two cycles (the first dose was administered on days 1 and 2 of the first cycle), every two weeks for cycles 3–6, and every month thereafter, Carfilzomib, twice per week at 20 mg/m^2 on days 1 and 2 of cycle 1 and at 56 mg/m^2 thereafter and dexamethasone 40 mg every week (20 mg for patients 75 years or older). After an initial follow up of 17 months, median PFS was not reached in the DKd group versus 15.8 months in the Kd group (HR 0.63; 95% CI 0.46–0.85; two-sided p = 0.0027) [34]. Data presented in the last ASH meeting showed further improvement in PFS for patients in the KRd arm. After 28 months of follow-up, the median PFS for KRd and Kd group were 28.6 and 15.2 months, respectively (HR, 0.59, 95% CI, 0.45–0.78]. PFS benefit was consistent among subgroups, especially in Lenalidomide refractory patients. Additionally, the MRD negativity rate at 12 months was significantly better in the DKd arm at 12.5% vs. 1.3% P < 0.0001. No new safety alerts have emerged [35].

2.2 Isatuximab

2.2.1 Mechanism of action

Isatuximab (SAR650984) is another chimeric IgG1κ monoclonal antibody, which binds on human CD38 by targeting a different epitope in comparison with Daratumumab [36]. Isatuximab and Daratumumab have several differences regarding the mechanism of action. 1/Isatuximab anti-tumor activity is mainly dependent on ADCC [37, 38] 2/Isatuximab induces direct apoptosis of CD-38 even in the absence of cross-linking agents [39] 3/Isatuximab inhibits CD-38 enzymatic activity in a dose-dependent manner [40].

2.2.2 Isatuximab clinical trials

In a phase I dose-escalation study, 84 patients with RRMM (median 5, range 1–13 prior lines of therapy) received Isatuximab monotherapy. Isatuximab administration showed clinical activity and a manageable safety profile. ORR was 24%, median PFS was 3.7 months. IRRs were mainly grade 1 or 2 that occurred during the first cycle [40]. These results were confirmed in a dose-finding phase II trial. Patients with RRMM who had received three or more prior lines of therapy were allocated to four different dosing schedules of isatuximab monotherapy: 3 mg/kg or 10 mg/kg every two weeks, 10 mg/kg every two weeks for one month and every month thereafter, and 20 mg/kg every week for one month and every two weeks thereafter. At doses ≥10 mg/kg 10 mg/kg OS and PFS were 18.7 and 4.6 months respectively, whereas ORR was 24.3% [41]. During the second part of the same study, patients with RRMM (median 4, range 2–10 prior lines of therapy) were randomized to receive isatuximab 20 mg/kg every week for one month, followed by 20 mg/kg every two weeks, with (n = 109) or without (n = 55) dexamethasone. Median PFS and OS were 4.9 and 18.9 and 10.2 for Isatuximab monotherapy and 10.2 and 17.3 for Isatuximab DEX group, respectively [42].

Isatuximab has also shown a synergistic effect when combined with Lenalidomide and dexamethasone. Fifty-seven patients with RRMM (median 5, range 1–12 prior lines of therapy) with 83% refractory to Lenalidomide received Isatuximab in combination with Lenalidomide and dexamethasone in this phase Ib dose-escalation study. The primary objective of the study was the determination of maximum tolerated dose (MTD) of Isatuximabwithin the combination with Lenalidomide and dexamethasone. The ORR was similar in both cohorts, 56%. Only one dose-limiting toxicity was reported (pneumonia grade II at 20 mg/kg/QW/Q2W), which resolved after discontinuation of treatment. The MTD was not reached. IRRs occurred mostly during the first infusion and were mild (grade I or II) regarding severity. These results demonstrate that the combination of Isatuximab with standard doses of Lenalidomide and Dexamethasone was active and well-tolerated in patients with RRMM [43].

Another phase Ib trial (NCT02283775) evaluated the tolerability and safety of Isatuximab in combination with Pomalidomide and low-dose dexamethasone in patients with RRMM, who had received prior treatment with a PI and Lenalidomide. Forty-five patients with a median of three (range 1–10) prior lines of therapy were recruited. 91% of patients were refractory to their last line of therapy, 84% were PI refractory, and 82% Lenalidomide refractory. Patients received Isatuximab at 5, 10, or 20 mg/kg (every week for four weeks and every two weeks thereafter), Pomalidomide 4 mg (days 1–21), and dexamethasone 40 mg weekly, in 28-days cycles until progressive disease or unacceptable toxicity. The primary objective was the determination of the recommended dose of Isatuximab within this combination, along with safety. Secondary objectives included evaluation of efficacy, pharmacokinetics, and immunogenicity. Among 45 enrolled patients, 8 received Isatuximab at 5 mg/kg, 31 at 10 mg/kg and 6 at 20 mg/kg for median duration of 9.6 months. The most common adverse events included fatigue (62%), infusion reactions (42%), and upper respiratory tract infections. Infusion-related reactions, which were mainly grade I or II, occurred mostly during the first administration of the drug and were manageable with corticosteroids and antihistamines. Median PFS and median duration of response were 17.6 and 18.7 months, respectively. ORR was 62%. These results demonstrated that the combination of Isatuximab with Pomalidomide and dexamethasone was safe and effective in heavily pretreated patients with MM [44].

Based on these encouraging results, the phase III ICARIA trial (NCT02990338) compared the combination Of Isatuximab Pom Dex (IPd) versus Pom dex (Pd) in 307 patients with RRMM who had received at least two prior lines of treatment, including Lenalidomide and a proteasome inhibitor (median three range 2–4). Patients received Isatuximab 10 mg/kg every week for the first cycle and on days 1 and 15 in the subsequent cycles, plus pomalidomide 4 mg/day (day 1–21) and dexamethasone 40 mg (or 20 mg for patients >75 years) weekly on 28 days cycles. Progression-free survival was the primary endpoint. After a median follow-up of 11.6 months, median progression-free survival was 11.5 months (95% CI 8.9–13.9) in the IPd group versus 6.5 months (4.5–8.3) in the Pd group;(HR 0.596, 95% CI 0.44–0.81; p = 0·001). Responses in the IPd arm occurred faster with a significantly longer duration in comparison with the IPd arm. Additionally, patients in the IPd arm achieved a higher percentage of MRD negativity. The addition of Isatuximab to Pom dex, resulted in significant improvement of PFS [45]. The consistency of the results from the primary analysis was evaluated in patients with soft tissue plasmacytomas. Data presented at the last ASH meeting showed that PFS and ORR were improved from the addition of Isatuximab to Pd in the subgroup of patients with extramedullary disease. Median PFS was 4.57 (95% CI: 2.40, not calculable) vs. 1.56 (95% CI: 0.95, 4.47) months in the IPd and Pd arm, respectively, whereas ORR was 50% (7/14 responders) and 10% (1/10 responders) in the IPd and Pd group. ASH 2289 Based on the results of the ICARIA trial, FDA and EMA approved the combination of IPd, in patients with RRMM.

The combination of Isatuximab with Carfilzomib has been evaluated in a phase Ib clinical trial (NCT02332850) [46]. In the dose-escalation part of the study, patients with RRMM who had received at least two prior (median three range 2–8) lines of treatment were randomized to receive Isatuximab in 3 different dose levels (DL) 10/kg every two weeks, 10 mg/kg every week for a month and every two weeks thereafter and 20 mg/kg every week for a month and every two weeks thereafter, in combination with K at dose 27 mg/m ^{2}. Fifteen patients received treatment in the dose-escalation and 18 in the dose-expansion cohort at DL2. The primary objective was the determination of the maximum tolerated dose (MTD). Secondary objectives included the assessment of efficacy and safety. Preliminary results showed a 66% ORR in all dose levels. Median PFS was not reached. Based on these results, the phase III IKEMA study (NCT03275285) compared the combination of IKd vs. Kd in the RR setting. Three hundred two patients with RRMM were randomized to receive IKd (n = 179) or Kd (n = 123). The administration of Isatuximab was 10 mg/kg iv weekly during the first month and every two weeks thereafter, whereas administration of Carfilzomib was 20 mg/m2 and 56 mg/m2 thereafter. The primary endpoint was PFS, and the secondary endpoints were OS and ORR [47]. Preliminary data were presented in the last ASH meeting. After a median follow-up of 20.7 months there was a statistically significant improvement of PFS in the IKd group (median PFS was not reached for IKd vs. 19.15 months for Kd; HR 0.531 (99% CI 0.318–0.889), one-sided p = 0.0007, with consistency among subgroups. ORR was 86.6% IKd vs. 82.9% for Kd, one-sided p = 0.1930. MRD negativity (10–5) in the intent to treat population (ITT) was 29.6% (53/179) vs. 13.0% (16/123) in the IKd and Kd groups, respectively descriptive p = 0.0004. Data regarding OS were immature at the time of primary analysis. The percentages of AES and SAEs were similar between the two groups. To conclude, the addition of Isatuximab to Kd lead to a significant improvement in PFS and depth of response. IKD may represent a new standard of care regimen for patients with RRMM [48].

Isatuximab is currently under investigation in the upfront setting. In transplant-ineligible patients, IMROZ trial (NCT03319667) is comparing the quadruplet combination Isatuximab-VRd with VRD, while another ongoing trial is comparing

Isatuximab-VRd to Isatuximab VCD(NCT02513186). In transplant-eligible patients, ISKIA trial is currently investigating the combination of Isatuximab-KRd vs. KRd as part of induction and consolidation regimen (NCT04483739).

2.3 Elotuzumab

2.3.1 Elotuzumab mechanism of action

SLAMF7 (signaling lymphocytic activation molecule family 7) or CD319 is a cell surface glycoprotein CD2/subset 1 (CS1). SLAMF7 expression is restricted to normal and abnormal plasma cells and NK lymphocytes [49]. Activation of SLAMf7 pathway promotes cell growth and survival. It also plays a critical role in the interaction with the bone marrow microenvironment [49, 50]. Elotuzumab is humanized, first in class IgG1 monoclonal antibody targeting SLAMF7. Elotuzumab primarily activates NK cells promoting antibody-dependent cellular cytotoxicity (ADCC). Elotuzumab has shown no activity when used as a single agent in MM patients.

2.3.2 Elotuzumab clinical trials

The large phase III ELOQUENT 2 trial (NCT01239797) evaluated the addition of Elotuzumab at the dose of 10 mg/kg to Lenalidomide and dexamethasone (Rd) in 646 patients with RRMM (94% lenalidomide naïve patients) who had received 1–3 prior lines of treatment. Patients received Lenalidomide 25 mg for days 1–21 and dexamethasone 40 mg on a weekly basis on 28-day cycles. Elotuzumab administration was 10 mg/kg weekly for the first two cycles, and 20 mg/kg on a monthly basis thereafter. Primary endpoints included PFS and ORR. OS was one of the key secondary endpoints. After an initial follow-up of 24.5 months, the rates of median PFS and ORR were 19.4 versus 14.9 months (HR for progression or death 0.70; 95% CI 0.57 to 0.85; $P < 0.001$) and 79%, versus 66% in the ELO Rd. and Rd. groups respectively. 26035255. PFS rates demonstrate sustained improvement after two (52%) and three (44%) years of follow-up (relative risk of disease progression or death by 30% and 27% respectively) 30204239. More recent data, after a 4-year follow-up, demonstrate sustained OS benefit (50 months for ELO Rd. versus 43 months for Rd. HR: 0.78; 95%CI: 0.63–0.96). 30719202 Administration of Elotuzumab was relatively safe. Most common grade 3 or 4 AEs in both arms included lymphopenia, neutropenia, pneumonia, and fatigue. Based on this trial Elotuzumab was granted approval by the FDA in December 2015 and EMA in 2016, in combination with Rd., for patients with RRMM, who had received at least one prior line of treatment [51].

Elotuzumab has also been evaluated in combination with Pomalidomide and dexamethasone (Pd). Eloquent 3 (NCT02654132) is a randomized phase II trial, comparing the combination of ELO Pd versus Pd in 117 patients who were refractory or relapsed and refractory to Lenalidomide and a proteasome inhibitor. Patients received Pomalidomide 4 mg for day 1–21 and dexamethasone 40 mg on a weekly basis on 28-day cycles. Elotuzumab administration was 10 mg/kg weekly for the first two cycles and 20 mg/kg on a monthly basis thereafter. Sixty patients were assigned to the ELO Pd group and 57 patients to the Pd group. After a follow up of 9.1 months, patients in the ELO Pd group had significantly increased PFS (10.3 vs. 4.7 months HR 0.54 CI0.34 to 0.86; $P = 0.008$) and ORR (53% vs. 26% odds ratio, 3.25; 95% CI, 1.49 to 7.11) in comparison with the Pd group. No significant differences were reported in the safety profiles of the two arms. Based on the results of the ELOQUENT III trial, Elotuzumab granted approval by the FDA in 2018 for RR patients who had received at least two prior lines of treatment, including Lenalidomide and a PI [52].

2.4 Antibody drug conjugates (ADCs)

BCMA, is a and member of the tumor necrosis factor receptors (TNFR) superfamily [53, 54]. BCMA is primarily expressed in late-stage B-lineage cells, normal and malignant plasma cells, and B-lymphocytes, with very low expression on non-hematologic cells [55]. BCMA has two main ligands: a proliferation-inducing ligand (APRIL) and B-cell activating factor (BAFF) [56–58]. Following binding of APRIL and BAFF, BCMA expression is selectively upregulated during malignant transformation of plasma cells, playing a critical role in survival, drug resistance, and tumor cell growth through activation of intracellular signal transduction pathways such as STAT3, phosphoinositide 3-kinase (PI3K), AKT, NFB and MAPK [59–63]. As demonstrated in BCMA knock-down mouse models, BCMA is not required for normal B-cell differentiation and homeostasis [64]. The shedding of BCMA from the cell surface is mediated by γ-secretase and results in a soluble form (soluble BCMA, sBCMA). Higher sBCMA levels have been associated with inferior clinical outcomes. In preclinical models, inhibition of BCMA, with specific antibodies, showed significant anti-myeloma activity. The aforementioned facts make BCMA an ideal therapeutic target for the treatment of Multiple Myeloma and provide the rationale for the development of anti-BCMA monoclonal antibodies.

GSK2857916 (Belantamab Mafodotin) is the first anti-BCMA ADC that has been investigated in clinical trials. This afucosylated, humanized, IgG1 monoclonal antibody is conjugated to monomethyl auristatin F (MMAF), an inhibitor of tubulin polymerization, through a protease-resistant maleimidocaproyl linker. Following binding to the plasma cell surface, GSK2857916 is internalized and the active cytotoxic drug (cys-mcMMAF) is released following enzymatic cleavage leading to cell death. Mechanisms of action include NK-cell mediated ADCC and ADCP [65].

DREAMM 1 (NCT02064387) is a first in human phase I, open-label study, which evaluated the administration of GSK2857916 in patients with RRMM and other hematologic malignancies expressing BCMA in terms of efficacy and safety. Dose escalation cohort (part I) included solely patients with MM who have failed previous treatment regimens, including stem cell transplant (if eligible) IMiDs, PIs, and alkylators, while the dose-expansion cohort (part2) included both patients with MM and relapsed follicular lymphoma or diffuse large B-cell lymphoma. Regarding MM patients in the expansion cohort, 57% had five or more prior lines of therapy; 89% were double (PI and IMiD) and 34% triple (PI, IMiD, and daratumumab) refractory. GSK2857916 was administered intravenously every three weeks as a 1 hr. infusion in 38 patients at different dose levels (0.03–4.6 mg/kg). Primary endpoints were safety, determination of maximum tolerated dose (MTD), and recommended phase 2 dose. Secondary objectives were the determination of pharmacodynamics and pharmacokinetics parameters, anti-drug antibodies, and clinical activity. In dose-expansion, patients received the selected recommended phase 2 dose of 3.4 mg/kg. Overall, 73 patients were recruited, thirty-eight in dose escalation and thirty-five in the dose-expansion cohort. Notably, BCMA expression was not included in the eligibility criteria of study [66].

Updated results of this study, after an extended median follow-up of 12.5 months, demonstrate that was effective in this heavily pretreated group of patients [67]. Achievement of response occurred early during the study after the first or second infusion. Interestingly, dose reduction did not affect the depth and duration of response. 21/65 patients in the dose-expansion part achieve partial or better response, including 2PRs, 14VGPRs, 3CRs, and two sCRs. 18/32 (56.3%)

patients who were double refractory (IMiDs and PIs) achieved response to treatment. For double refractory patients (IMiDs and PIs), with prior Daratumumab exposure, OR was 38.5%. The median PFS and DOR were 12 and 14.3 months, respectively. Among double refractory patients, the median PFS was 7.9 months. For patients with and without prior Daratumumab exposure, median PFS was 6.8 and 15.7 months, respectively. For double refractory patients with prior Daratumumab exposure, median PFS was 6.2 months [67].

The most frequent AEs were fatigue, nausea, chills, anemia, pyrexia, hypercalcemia, thrombocytopenia, and dry eye, while the most common grade 3 or 4 toxicities included neutropenia, anemia, and thrombocytopenia. Infusion-related reactions (IRRs) (Grade 1 or 2) were reported in 7 patients across all dose levels, and all of them occurred during the first dose. Of note, there were no dose-limiting toxicities (DLT) and no MTD identified in the dose-escalation phase. Ocular toxicity, including blurred vision, foreign body sensation, and photophobia, were common presented in 53% of patients in part 1 and in 63% in part 2. Most common findings during eye examination under a slim lamp included keratitis and corneal microcystic changes. All AEs were reversible. The median time to onset was 23 days (range 1–84). Management included dose reductions and/or delays, artificial tears, and steroid eye drops. The median time to resolution was 30 days (range 5–224). Even though the exact pathophysiologic mechanism of keratopathy is unknown, it may be attributed to the uptake of the payload (MMAF) in the basal epithelial layer of the cornea 2938270. Ocular toxicity resulted in two treatment discontinuations in part 1 and no discontinuations in part 2 of the study. The main reasons for treatment discontinuation were disease progression (n = 15) and AEs (n = 2). Based on these promising results, FDA granted GSK2857916 a breakthrough therapy designation for the treatment of RRMM patients who had receive three prior lines of treatment, including an anti-CD38 antibody, and were refractory to both an IMiD and a PI [68].

Following the encouraging results of DREAMM-1 study, the subsequent DREAMM-2 trial (NCT03525678) further explored the safety and activity of Belantamab mafodotin (GSK2857916) in the RR setting. Patients were refractory to PI, IMiD and an anti-CD38 mAb alone or in combination and randomized 1:1 to receive 2.5 mg/kg (n = 97) or 3.4 mg/kg (n = 99) Belantamab Mafodotin iv, every three weeks until disease progression or unacceptable toxicity. Regarding refractoriness to previous lines of treatment, 76% and 75% were refractory to bortezomib, 65% and 58% to Carfilzomib, 90% and 89% to Lenalidomide, 87% and 78% to Pomalidomide and 100% and 92% to Daratumumab in the 2.5 and 3.4 mg/kg dose arms, respectively. Patients had receive a median of 6 (range 3–21) and 7(range 3–21) prior lines of treatment, respectively [69].

Overall response rate (ORR) was the primary objective of the study. After a median follow up of 6.5 months (6.3 in the 2.5 mg cohort and 6.9 in the 3.4 mg cohort), median PFS was 2.9(95% CI: 2.1–3.7) and 4.9(95% CI: 2.3–6.2) months in the two groups while the ORR was 31% (30/97 97.5% CI 20.8–42.6) and 34% (34/99CI 23.9–46) respectively 31859245. At this time point, OS data were not mature. Updated analysis of this trial, with a median, follow up of 9 months, demonstrated a median PFS of 2.8 and 3.9 months in the two cohorts with one year OS probability of 53% 21/48 and similar ORR among the group of patients with 3–6 (34%) and seven or more (30%) prior lines of therapy [69]. Two post hoc analyses demonstrate the efficacy of Belantamab mafodotin in the subgroups of patients with high-risk cytogenetics and impaired renal function (EGFR 30 ml/min) [70, 71].

Regarding AEs, this study confirmed the frequent occurrence of corneal events. 72% of patients developed keratopathy of any grade, while 31% developed keratopathy grade 3–4. Keratopathy was attributed to the MMAF payload and was reversible after temporary discontinuation of the drug. Other frequent adverse events grade 3–4 were anemia (21%) and thrombocytopenia (22%). Infusion-related reactions (IRRs) were reported in 21% and 16% in the two treatment arms and were mostly grade 1 or 2. Serious AEs occurred in 40% and 47% in the 2.5 mg/kg and 3.4 mg/kg cohorts respectively. Two reported cases lead to death, potentially connected to study drug. One case of sepsis in the 2.5 mg/kg and one of haemophagocytic lymphohistiocytosis in the 3.4 mg/kg cohort.

Currently, the role of Belantamab Mafodotin (GSK2857916) is being evaluated in the RRMM setting.

DREAMM-6 (NCT03544281) is an ongoing Phase I/II, a two-part study of GSK2857916 in combination with lenalidomide/dexamethasone (Arm A) or BorDex (Arm B) in patients with RRMM who had received ≥one prior therapy. Refractory to Bortezomib patients were not excluded. Preliminary results from Arm B, presented in the last ASH meeting, have shown a high ORR of 78% (95% CI 52.4–93.6). No new safety signals have emerged.

Three-phase III studies are currently ongoing, evaluating the safety and efficacy of belantamab mafodotin in combination with Pomalidomide (NCT04162210; DREAMM-3) daratumumab plus bortezomib (NCT04246047; DREAMM-7) or Pomalidomide plus Bortezomib (NCT04484623: DREAMM-8). The results are eagerly awaited.

MEDI2228 is another antibody-drug conjugate (ADC) composed of fully human monoclonal antibody, conjugated to a dimeric cross-linking pyrrolobenzodiazepine (PBD) dimer (tesirine) via a protease-cleavable dipeptide (valine-alanine) linker8/42 MEDI2228 has shown potent antitumor activity in preclinical models, including cell lines resistant to Lenalidomide. Based on these reports, a phase I open-label, dose-escalation, and expansion first in-human study (NCT03489525) evaluated safety, clinical activity, and pharmacokinetics of MEDI2228 in patients with RRMM. All patients had progressive disease after treatment with an IMiD, a PI, and a monoclonal antibody. In the dose-escalation part of the study, MEDI2228 was administered iv every three weeks in five sequentially ascending dose levels (0.0125, 0.025, 0.05, 0.1, and 0.2 mg/kg). DLTS lead to dose de-escalation from 0.2 mg/kg to 0.14 mg/kg. Primary endpoints included safety and tolerability. 0.14 mg/kg Q3W was determined as the maximum tolerated dose (MTD). In the 0.14 mg/kg cohort 53.7% experienced photophobia and 19.5% eye dryness. There were no incidents of visual acuity loss or keratopathy in the 0.14 mg/kg cohort. Other treatment-related AEs included thrombocytopenia (31.7%) rash (29.3%), increased gamma-glutamyltransferase (24.4%) and pleural effusion (19.5%). In the 0.14 mg/kg cohort, ORR was 61.0% (95% [CI]: 44.5%, 75.8%), including 10 (24.4%) VGPRs and 15 (36.6%) PR. These data suggest that MEDI2228 is clinically efficient in this heavily pretreated group of patients [72].

2.5 Bispecific antibodies

Bispecific T-cell engagers (BiTEs) are monoclonal antibodies with two separate antigen recognition domains. One with a high affinity to an antigen in the surface of tumor cell and another targeting CD-3 in the surface of T-cells. Binding to those two distinct epitopes leads to the formation of an immunologic synapse. Binding to the CD3e epitope augments the t-cell recruitment and activation, leading to cell death. In MM, the majority of BiTEs targeting BCMA in the surface of plasma cells.

AMG-420, formerly known as BI 836909, is the first BiTE demonstrating clinical activity. It is comprised of two single-chain variable fragments (scFvs), one targeting BCMA and one targeting CD3. AMG-420 is the compound with the most available data to date. In a first in human dose-escalation study, AMG420 was administered in 42 patients with RRMM (NCT02514239). Eligible patients had progressed after a minimum of 2 prior lines of treatment, including a PI and an IMiD 31895611. The median number of prior lines of therapy was 4 (range 2–13). 31% of patients were double refractory to IMiDs and PIs, and 21% were daratumumab refractory. AMG420 was administered at different dose levels, 0.2-800 μg/d, through a continuous iv infusion for four weeks in 6-week cycles due to its low molecular weight and short half-life. Patients received treatment for up to 10 cycles Monitoring of toxicities required hospitalization at the beginning of cycles one (4 days) and two (1 day) [73].

There were two deaths reported from adverse events: One patient in the 50 μg/d cohort died after the first cycle due to respiratory distress syndrome caused by concurrent influenza and aspergillosis, and one from hepatic failure from adenovirus. None of these incidents were considered related to treatment. There were no grade 3 or greater CNS toxicities reported. At the 800 μg/d dose level, two-thirds of the patients experienced DLTs. One patient had gr 3 CRS and one gr 3 peripheral polyneuropathy, which included progressive dysfunction of the peripheral motor and sensory nerves. Following the interruption of the study drug, both toxicities resolved. No DLTs were observed up to the level of 400 μg/d. In the most recent follow-up of the study, 40 patients discontinued treatment. Twenty-five due to disease progression, seven due to AEs, four died, three completed treatment (10 cycles), and 1 withdraw consent [73]. ORR was 31% (13/42patients). At the MTD of 400 μg/d, the response rate was 70% (7/10). In the 400 μg/d group, five patients achieved MRD negativity, one achieved PR, and one VGPR.

As mentioned, because of its low molecular weight and short half-life, AMG420 was administered through a continuous iv infusion for four weeks in 6-week cycles due to its low molecular weight and short half-life. AMG 701, a BiTE with an extended half-life allowing once-weekly subcutaneous administration, was developed and is currently under investigation (NCT03287908).

PF-06863135 (PF-3135) is a humanized Ig-like Bispecific antibody targeting both BCMA and CD3. PF-06863135 has been administered intravenously at 0.1–50 μg/kg weekly in patients with RRMM. Preliminary results demonstrate antimyeloma activity. The maximum tolerated dose was not reached [74]. In order to reduce the maximum concentration (Cmax) of the drug, which was possibly associated with inflammatory response and cytokine release syndrome (CRS), subcutaneous administration of the drug was tested. Preliminary results were reported in the last ASH meeting [75]. 2 6/8(75%) patients achieved a response at the two highest dose levels evaluated. The sc administration modulates Cmax. This could allow the administration of higher doses without increased incidence of CRS. The trial is ongoing.

3. Immune checkpoint inhibitors

The programmed death-1 (PD-1) receptor is a type-1 transmembrane glycoprotein, expressed on antigen-activated B-cells, T-cells, and NK-cells. The binding of PD-1 ligands (PD-L1 and PD-L2) on PD-1 receptor results in downregulation of immune functions mediated by T-cells such as cytokine production, t-cell proliferation, and cytotoxicity [76]. The overexpression of PD-L1 and PD-L2 is a well recognizable mechanism of immune evasion. Preclinical data from MM patients have shown an increased expression of PD-L1 and PD-1 on malignant plasma cells and T and NK cells respectively [77, 78]. The deciphering of this particular mechanism of action has lead to the development of immune checkpoint inhibitors that

Description	Phase	NCT number	Population
DARATUMUMAB			
A Study of Daratumumab Plus Lenalidomide Versus Lenalidomide Alone as Maintenance Treatment in Participants With Newly Diagnosed Multiple Myeloma Who Are Minimal Residual Disease Positive After Frontline Autologous Stem Cell Transplant (AURIGA)	3	NCT03901963	NDMM
Study of Melphalan Flufenamide (Melflufen) in Combination With Daratumumab in Relapsed Refractory Multiple Myeloma (LIGHTHOUSE)	3	NCT04649060	RRMM
Daratumumab, VELCADE (Bortezomib), Lenalidomide and Dexamethasone Compared to VELCADE, Lenalidomide and Dexamethasone in Subjects With Previously Untreated Multiple Myeloma (PERSEUS)	3	NCT03710603	NDMM
ISATUXIMAB			
Isatuximab Bortezomib, Lenalidomide and Dexamethasone Combination in NDMM Patients Not Eligible for Transplant (IMROZ)	3	NCT03319667	NDMM
Isa-KRd vs. KRd in Newly Diagnosed Multiple Myeloma Patients Eligible for Autologous Stem Cell Transplantation (IsKia)	3	NCT04483739	NDMM
ANTIBODY-DRUG CONJUGATES			
Study of Single Agent Belantamab Mafodotin Versus Pomalidomide Plus Low-dose Dexamethasone (Pom/Dex) in Participants With Relapsed/Refractory Multiple Myeloma (DREAMM-3)	3	NCT04162210	RRMM
Study Evaluating Safety, Tolerability and Clinical Activity of GSK2857916 in Combination With Pembrolizumab in Subjects With Relapsed/Refractory Multiple Myeloma (DREAMM-4)	1/2	NCT03848845	RRMM
Platform Study of Belantamab Mafodotin as Monotherapy and in Combination With Anti-cancer Treatments in Participants With Relapsed/Refractory Multiple Myeloma (RRMM) (DREAMM 5)	1/2	NCT04126200	RRMM
To Evaluate Safety, Tolerability, and Clinical Activity of the Antibody-drug Conjugate, GSK2857916 Administered in Combination With Lenalidomide Plus Dexamethasone (Arm A), or in Combination With Bortezomib Plus Dexamethasone (Arm B) in Participants With Relapsed/Refractory Multiple Myeloma (DREAMM-6)	1/2	NCT03544281	RRMM
Evaluation of Efficacy and Safety of Belantamab Mafodotin, Bortezomib and Dexamethasone Versus Daratumumab, Bortezomib and Dexamethasone in Participants With Relapsed/Refractory Multiple Myeloma (DREAMM-7)	3	NCT04246047	RRMM
Belantamab Mafodotin Plus Pomalidomide and Dexamethasone (Pd) Versus Bortezomib Plus Pd in Relapsed/Refractory Multiple Myeloma (DREAMM-8)	3	NCT04484623	RRMM
Study of Belantamab Mafodotin Plus Standard of Care (SoC) in Newly Diagnosed Multiple Myeloma (DREAMM-9)	1	NCT04091126	NDMM

Description	Phase	NCT number	Population
A Study of Belantamab Mafodotin (GSK2857916) in Multiple Myeloma Participants With Normal and Varying Degree of Impaired Renal Function (DREAMM-12)	1	NCT04398745	RRMM
A Study of Belantamab Mafodotin (GSK2857916) in Multiple Myeloma Participants With Normal and Impaired Hepatic Function (DREAMM-13)	1	NCT04398680	RRMM
BISPECIFIC ANTIBODIES			
PF-06863135 As Single Agent And In Combination With Immunomodulatory Agents In Relapse/ Refractory Multiple Myeloma	1	NCT03269136	RRMM
MagnetisMM-3: Study Of Elranatamab (PF-06863135) Monotherapy in Participants With Multiple Myeloma Who Are Refractory to at Least One PI, One IMiD and One Anti-CD38 mAb	2	NCT04649359	RRMM
First in Human (FIH) Study of REGN5458 in Patients With Relapsed or Refractory Multiple Myeloma	1/2	NCT03761108	RRMM
A Study of Teclistamab, in Participants With Relapsed or Refractory Multiple Myeloma	2	NCT04557098	RRMM
A Study of Talquetamab in Participants With Relapsed or Refractory Multiple Myeloma	2	NCT04634552	RRMM

Table 1.
Ongoing clinical trials.

block receptors (PD-1) and ligands (PD-L1 and PD-L2), resulting in the recovery of immune response.

Pembrolizumab is a humanized IgG4 monoclonal antibody with high specificity against PD-1 receptors. Pembrolizumab was evaluated in combination with Lenalidomide and low dose dexamethasone in a phase I dose-escalation study (KEYNOTE-023 trial NCT02036502). Sixty-six patients with RRMM were recruited. Pembrolizumab was treatment-related AEs. Grade 3 AEs (mainly cytopenias fatigue and diarrhea) occurred in 37 (59,7%) patients. ORR OS and median PFS were 44%, not reached, and 7.2 months respectively [79, 80]. Pembrolizumab has also been evaluated in combination with Pomalidomide and dexamethasone in another phase II study (NCT02289222). Forty-eight patients with RRMM were recruited. Patients had received 2–5 (median 3) prior lines of treatment. 73% were refractory to both IMIDs and PIs. ORR was 60%. The percentage of SCR and CR, VGPR, and PR were 8%, 19%, and 33%, respectively. After a median follow-up of 15.6 months, OS and PFS were not reached and 17.4 months, respectively. (40%) [81].

Based on these results, two-phase three trials were designed to evaluate the combination of Pembrolizumab dexamethasone with Lenalidomide (KEYNOTE-185 NCT02579863) or Pomalidomide (KEYNOTE-183 NCT02576977) in ND and RR setting respectively. Interim analysis of both studies showed excessive administered for a median of 7 cycles (range 1–67). Overall, 95% of patients experienced unanticipated deaths attributed to the combination of Pembrolizumab Dexamethasone with Lenalidomide or Pomalidomide. These results showed that the risk profile of these novel combinations was unfavorable, and both trials were terminated early [82, 83].

Nivolumab is a fully human IgG4 Moab targeting PD-1 receptors. Investigation of Nivolumab with IMiDS has been placed on clinical hold after reviewing data regarding Pembrolizumab. Nivolumab is currently under investigation in combination with daratumumab (NCT03184194), Elotuzumab (NCT02612779), Pomalidomide (NCT02726581), and Carfilzomib (NCT03605719) in phase 2 trials.

In **Table 1**, we present selected clinical trials conducted with monoclonal antibodies in the newly diagnosed and relapsed refractory setting.

4. Conclusion

Despite therapeutic improvements Multiple Myeloma remain an incurable disease. The treatment of patients with RR remains a challenging issue. Antibody therapy has significantly enhanced the armamentarium of therapeutic options. Further research should focus on tailoring the combination regimens based on disease and patient characteristics in order to optimize the efficacy and safety.

Author details

Nikolaos Kanellias*, Maria Gavriatopoulou and Evangelos Terpos
Department of Clinical Therapeutics, Medical School, Alexandra General Hospital, National and Kapodistrian University of Athens, Athens, Greece

*Address all correspondence to: nick.kanellias@gmail.com

References

[1] Palumbo A, Anderson K. Multiple myeloma. N Engl J Med 2011; 364: 1046-1060.

[2] Kumar SK, Lee JH, Lahuerta JJ et al. Risk of progression and survival in multiple myeloma relapsing after therapy with IMiDs and bortezomib: a multicenter international myeloma working group study. Leukemia 2012; 26: 149-157.

[3] Kumar SK, Dimopoulos MA, Kastritis E et al. Natural history of relapsed myeloma, refractory to immunomodulatory drugs and proteasome inhibitors: a multicenter IMWG study. Leukemia 2017; 31: 2443-2448.

[4] van de Donk NW, Sonneveld P. Diagnosis and risk stratification in multiple myeloma. Hematol Oncol Clin North Am 2014; 28: 791-813.

[5] Sonneveld P, Avet-Loiseau H, Lonial S et al. Treatment of multiple myeloma with high-risk cytogenetics: a consensus of the International Myeloma Working Group. Blood 2016; 127: 2955-2962.

[6] de Weers M, Tai YT, van der Veer MS et al. Daratumumab, a novel therapeutic human CD38 monoclonal antibody, induces killing of multiple myeloma and other hematological tumors. J Immunol 2011; 186: 1840-1848.

[7] Pelton JG, Wemmer DE. Structural modeling of the distamycin A-d(CGCGAATTCGCG)2 complex using 2D NMR and molecular mechanics. Biochemistry 1988; 27: 8088-8096.

[8] Overdijk MB, Verploegen S, Bogels M et al. Antibody-mediated phagocytosis contributes to the anti-tumor activity of the therapeutic antibody daratumumab in lymphoma and multiple myeloma. MAbs 2015; 7: 311-321.

[9] Phipps C, Chen Y, Gopalakrishnan S, Tan D. Daratumumab and its potential in the treatment of multiple myeloma: overview of the preclinical and clinical development. Ther Adv Hematol 2015; 6: 120-127.

[10] Jain A, Ramasamy K. Evolving Role of Daratumumab: From Backbencher to Frontline Agent. Clin Lymphoma Myeloma Leuk 2020; 20: 572-587.

[11] Bonello F, Mina R, Boccadoro M, Gay F. Therapeutic Monoclonal Antibodies and Antibody Products: Current Practices and Development in Multiple Myeloma. Cancers (Basel) 2019; 12.

[12] Krejcik J, Casneuf T, Nijhof IS et al. Daratumumab depletes CD38+ immune regulatory cells, promotes T-cell expansion, and skews T-cell repertoire in multiple myeloma. Blood 2016; 128: 384-394.

[13] van der Veer MS, de Weers M, van Kessel B et al. The therapeutic human CD38 antibody daratumumab improves the anti-myeloma effect of newly emerging multi-drug therapies. Blood Cancer J 2011; 1: e41.

[14] Usmani SZ, Weiss BM, Plesner T et al. Clinical efficacy of daratumumab monotherapy in patients with heavily pretreated relapsed or refractory multiple myeloma. Blood 2016; 128: 37-44.

[15] Dimopoulos MA, Oriol A, Nahi H et al. Daratumumab, Lenalidomide, and Dexamethasone for Multiple Myeloma. N Engl J Med 2016; 375: 1319-1331.

[16] Chatterjee S, Daenthanasanmak A, Chakraborty P et al. CD38-NAD(+)Axis Regulates Immunotherapeutic Anti-Tumor T Cell Response. Cell Metab 2018; 27: 85-100 e108.

[17] Mateos MV, Dimopoulos MA, Cavo M et al. Daratumumab plus Bortezomib, Melphalan, and Prednisone for Untreated Myeloma. N Engl J Med 2018; 378: 518-528.

[18] Terpos E, Ntanasis-Stathopoulos I, International Myeloma S. Clinical Updates Regarding Multiple Myeloma From the 2019 American Society of Hematology Annual Meeting. Clin Lymphoma Myeloma Leuk 2020; 20: 499-508.

[19] Mateos MV, Cavo M, Blade J et al. Overall survival with daratumumab, bortezomib, melphalan, and prednisone in newly diagnosed multiple myeloma (ALCYONE): a randomised, open-label, phase 3 trial. Lancet 2020; 395: 132-141.

[20] San-Miguel JF, Avet-Loiseau H, Paiva B et al. Sustained Minimal Residual Disease (MRD) Negativity and Clinical Efficacy in Transplant-Ineligible (TIE) Newly Diagnosed Multiple Myeloma (NDMM) Patients (Pts) Treated with Daratumumab-Based Regimens: Analysis of Maia and Alcyone. Blood 2020; 136: 18-20.

[21] Facon T, Kumar S, Plesner T et al. Daratumumab plus Lenalidomide and Dexamethasone for Untreated Myeloma. N Engl J Med 2019; 380: 2104-2115.

[22] Bahlis N, Facon T, Usmani SZ et al. Daratumumab Plus Lenalidomide and Dexamethasone (D-Rd) Versus Lenalidomide and Dexamethasone (Rd) in Patients with Newly Diagnosed Multiple Myeloma (NDMM) Ineligible for Transplant: Updated Analysis of Maia. Blood 2019; 134: 1875-1875.

[23] Kumar SK, Facon T, Usmani SZ et al. Updated Analysis of Daratumumab Plus Lenalidomide and Dexamethasone (D-Rd) Versus Lenalidomide and Dexamethasone (Rd) in Patients with Transplant-Ineligible Newly Diagnosed Multiple Myeloma (NDMM): The Phase 3 Maia Study. Blood 2020; 136: 24-26.

[24] Chari A, Martinez-Lopez J, Mateos M-V et al. Daratumumab plus carfilzomib and dexamethasone in patients with relapsed or refractory multiple myeloma. Blood 2019; 134: 421-431.

[25] Voorhees PM, Kaufman JL, Laubach J et al. Daratumumab, lenalidomide, bortezomib, and dexamethasone for transplant-eligible newly diagnosed multiple myeloma: the GRIFFIN trial. Blood 2020; 136: 936-945.

[26] Voorhees PM, Rodriguez C, Reeves B et al. Daratumumab plus RVd for newly diagnosed multiple myeloma: final analysis of the safety run-in cohort of GRIFFIN. Blood Advances 2021; 5: 1092-1096.

[27] Moreau P, Attal M, Hulin C et al. Bortezomib, thalidomide, and dexamethasone with or without daratumumab before and after autologous stem-cell transplantation for newly diagnosed multiple myeloma (CASSIOPEIA): a randomised, open-label, phase 3 study. Lancet 2019; 394: 29-38.

[28] Costa LJ, Chhabra S, Godby KN et al. Daratumumab, Carfilzomib, Lenalidomide and Dexamethasone (Dara-KRd) Induction, Autologous Transplantation and Post-Transplant, Response-Adapted, Measurable Residual Disease (MRD)-Based Dara-Krd Consolidation in Patients with Newly Diagnosed Multiple Myeloma (NDMM). Blood 2019; 134: 860-860.

[29] Dimopoulos MA, San-Miguel J, Belch A et al. Daratumumab plus lenalidomide and dexamethasone versus lenalidomide and dexamethasone in relapsed or refractory multiple myeloma: updated analysis of POLLUX. Haematologica 2018; 103: 2088-2096.

[30] Bahlis NJ, Dimopoulos MA, White DJ et al. Daratumumab plus lenalidomide and dexamethasone in

relapsed/refractory multiple myeloma: extended follow-up of POLLUX, a randomized, open-label, phase 3 study. Leukemia 2020; 34: 1875-1884.

[31] Palumbo A, Chanan-Khan A, Weisel K et al. Daratumumab, Bortezomib, and Dexamethasone for Multiple Myeloma. N Engl J Med 2016; 375: 754-766.

[32] Chari A, Suvannasankha A, Fay JW et al. Daratumumab plus pomalidomide and dexamethasone in relapsed and/or refractory multiple myeloma. Blood 2017; 130: 974-981.

[33] Dimopoulos MA, Terpos E, Boccadoro M et al. Apollo: Phase 3 Randomized Study of Subcutaneous Daratumumab Plus Pomalidomide and Dexamethasone (D-Pd) Versus Pomalidomide and Dexamethasone (Pd) Alone in Patients (Pts) with Relapsed/Refractory Multiple Myeloma (RRMM). Blood 2020; 136: 5-6.

[34] Usmani SZ, Quach H, Mateos M-V et al. Carfilzomib, Dexamethasone, and Daratumumab Versus Carfilzomib and Dexamethasone for the Treatment of Patients with Relapsed or Refractory Multiple Myeloma (RRMM): Primary Analysis Results from the Randomized, Open-Label, Phase 3 Study Candor (NCT03158688). Blood 2019; 134: LBA-6-LBA-6.

[35] Dimopoulos MA, Quach H, Mateos M-V et al. Carfilzomib, Dexamethasone, and Daratumumab Versus Carfilzomib and Dexamethasone in Relapsed or Refractory Multiple Myeloma: Updated Efficacy and Safety Results of the Phase 3 Candor Study. Blood 2020; 136: 26-27.

[36] Deckert J, Wetzel MC, Bartle LM et al. SAR650984, a novel humanized CD38-targeting antibody, demonstrates potent antitumor activity in models of multiple myeloma and other CD38+ hematologic malignancies. Clin Cancer Res 2014; 20: 4574-4583.

[37] Nijhof IS, Groen RW, Noort WA et al. Preclinical Evidence for the Therapeutic Potential of CD38-Targeted Immuno-Chemotherapy in Multiple Myeloma Patients Refractory to Lenalidomide and Bortezomib. Clin Cancer Res 2015; 21: 2802-2810.

[38] van der Veer MS, de Weers M, van Kessel B et al. Towards effective immunotherapy of myeloma: enhanced elimination of myeloma cells by combination of lenalidomide with the human CD38 monoclonal antibody daratumumab. Haematologica 2011; 96: 284-290.

[39] Overdijk MB, Jansen JH, Nederend M et al. The Therapeutic CD38 Monoclonal Antibody Daratumumab Induces Programmed Cell Death via Fcgamma Receptor-Mediated Cross-Linking. J Immunol 2016; 197: 807-813.

[40] Martin T, Strickland S, Glenn M et al. Phase I trial of isatuximab monotherapy in the treatment of refractory multiple myeloma. Blood Cancer J 2019; 9: 41.

[41] Mikhael J, Richter J, Vij R et al. A dose-finding Phase 2 study of single agent isatuximab (anti-CD38 mAb) in relapsed/refractory multiple myeloma. Leukemia 2020; 34: 3298-3309.

[42] Dimopoulos M, Bringhen S, Anttila P et al. Isatuximab as monotherapy and combined with dexamethasone in patients with relapsed/refractory multiple myeloma. Blood 2021; 137: 1154-1165.

[43] Martin T, Baz R, Benson DM et al. A phase 1b study of isatuximab plus lenalidomide and dexamethasone for relapsed/refractory multiple myeloma. Blood 2017; 129: 3294-3303.

[44] Mikhael J, Richardson P, Usmani SZ et al. A phase 1b study of isatuximab plus pomalidomide/dexamethasone in relapsed/refractory multiple myeloma. Blood 2019; 134: 123-133.

[45] Attal M, Richardson PG, Rajkumar SV et al. Isatuximab plus pomalidomide and low-dose dexamethasone versus pomalidomide and low-dose dexamethasone in patients with relapsed and refractory multiple myeloma (ICARIA-MM): a randomised, multicentre, open-label, phase 3 study. Lancet 2019; 394: 2096-2107.

[46] Chari A, Richter JR, Shah N et al. Phase I-b study of isatuximab + carfilzomib in relapsed and refractory multiple myeloma (RRMM). Journal of Clinical Oncology 2018; 36: 8014-8014.

[47] Moreau P, Dimopoulos MA, Yong K et al. Isatuximab plus carfilzomib/dexamethasone versus carfilzomib/dexamethasone in patients with relapsed/refractory multiple myeloma: IKEMA Phase III study design. Future Oncol 2020; 16: 4347-4358.

[48] Martin T, Mikhael J, Hajek R et al. Depth of Response and Response Kinetics of Isatuximab Plus Carfilzomib and Dexamethasone in Relapsed Multiple Myeloma: Ikema Interim Analysis. Blood 2020; 136: 7-8.

[49] Tai YT, Dillon M, Song W et al. Anti-CS1 humanized monoclonal antibody HuLuc63 inhibits myeloma cell adhesion and induces antibody-dependent cellular cytotoxicity in the bone marrow milieu. Blood 2008; 112: 1329-1337.

[50] Pazina T, James AM, MacFarlane AWt et al. The anti-SLAMF7 antibody elotuzumab mediates NK cell activation through both CD16-dependent and -independent mechanisms. Oncoimmunology 2017; 6: e1339853.

[51] Lonial S, Dimopoulos M, Palumbo A et al. Elotuzumab Therapy for Relapsed or Refractory Multiple Myeloma. N Engl J Med 2015; 373: 621-631.

[52] Dimopoulos MA, Dytfeld D, Grosicki S et al. Elotuzumab plus Pomalidomide and Dexamethasone for Multiple Myeloma. N Engl J Med 2018; 379: 1811-1822.

[53] Madry C, Laabi Y, Callebaut I et al. The characterization of murine BCMA gene defines it as a new member of the tumor necrosis factor receptor superfamily. Int Immunol 1998; 10: 1693-1702.

[54] Sanchez E, Li M, Kitto A et al. Serum B-cell maturation antigen is elevated in multiple myeloma and correlates with disease status and survival. Br J Haematol 2012; 158: 727-738.

[55] Carpenter RO, Evbuomwan MO, Pittaluga S et al. B-cell maturation antigen is a promising target for adoptive T-cell therapy of multiple myeloma. Clin Cancer Res 2013; 19: 2048-2060.

[56] Thompson JS, Schneider P, Kalled SL et al. BAFF binds to the tumor necrosis factor receptor-like molecule B cell maturation antigen and is important for maintaining the peripheral B cell population. J Exp Med 2000; 192: 129-135.

[57] Novak AJ, Darce JR, Arendt BK et al. Expression of BCMA, TACI, and BAFF-R in multiple myeloma: a mechanism for growth and survival. Blood 2004; 103: 689-694.

[58] Gavriatopoulou M, Ntanasis-Stathopoulos I, Dimopoulos MA, Terpos E. Anti-BCMA antibodies in the future management of multiple myeloma. Expert Rev Anticancer Ther 2019; 19: 319-326.

[59] Shen X, Guo Y, Qi J et al. Binding of B-cell maturation antigen to B-cell activating factor induces survival of multiple myeloma cells by activating Akt and JNK signaling pathways. Cell Biochem Funct 2016; 34: 104-110.

[60] Demchenko YN, Kuehl WM. A critical role for the NFkB pathway in multiple myeloma. Oncotarget 2010; 1: 59-68.

[61] Chatterjee M, Jain S, Stuhmer T et al. STAT3 and MAPK signaling maintain overexpression of heat shock proteins 90alpha and beta in multiple myeloma cells, which critically contribute to tumor-cell survival. Blood 2007; 109: 720-728.

[62] Lentzsch S, Chatterjee M, Gries M et al. PI3-K/AKT/FKHR and MAPK signaling cascades are redundantly stimulated by a variety of cytokines and contribute independently to proliferation and survival of multiple myeloma cells. Leukemia 2004; 18: 1883-1890.

[63] Chatterjee M, Stuhmer T, Herrmann P et al. Combined disruption of both the MEK/ERK and the IL-6R/STAT3 pathways is required to induce apoptosis of multiple myeloma cells in the presence of bone marrow stromal cells. Blood 2004; 104: 3712-3721.

[64] O'Connor BP, Raman VS, Erickson LD et al. BCMA is essential for the survival of long-lived bone marrow plasma cells. J Exp Med 2004; 199: 91-98.

[65] Tai YT, Mayes PA, Acharya C et al. Novel anti-B-cell maturation antigen antibody-drug conjugate (GSK2857916) selectively induces killing of multiple myeloma. Blood 2014; 123: 3128-3138.

[66] Trudel S, Lendvai N, Popat R et al. Targeting B-cell maturation antigen with GSK2857916 antibody-drug conjugate in relapsed or refractory multiple myeloma (BMA117159): a dose escalation and expansion phase 1 trial. Lancet Oncol 2018; 19: 1641-1653.

[67] Trudel S, Lendvai N, Popat R et al. Antibody-drug conjugate, GSK2857916, in relapsed/refractory multiple myeloma: an update on safety and efficacy from dose expansion phase I study. Blood Cancer J 2019; 9: 37.

[68] Tzogani K, Penttila K, Lahteenvuo J et al. EMA Review of Belantamab Mafodotin (Blenrep) for the Treatment of Adult Patients with Relapsed/Refractory Multiple Myeloma. Oncologist 2021; 26: 70-76.

[69] Lonial S, Lee HC, Badros A et al. Belantamab mafodotin for relapsed or refractory multiple myeloma (DREAMM-2): a two-arm, randomised, open-label, phase 2 study. Lancet Oncol 2020; 21: 207-221.

[70] Cohen AD, Trudel S, Lonial S et al. DREAMM-2: Single-agent belantamab mafodotin (GSK2857916) in patients with relapsed/refractory multiple myeloma (RRMM) and high-risk (HR) cytogenetics. Journal of Clinical Oncology 2020; 38: 8541-8541.

[71] Lee HC, Cohen AD, Chari A et al. DREAMM-2: Single-agent belantamab mafodotin (GSK2857916) in patients with relapsed/refractory multiple myeloma (RRMM) and renal impairment. Journal of Clinical Oncology 2020; 38: 8519-8519.

[72] Kumar SK, Migkou M, Bhutani M et al. Phase 1, First-in-Human Study of MEDI2228, a BCMA-Targeted ADC in Patients with Relapsed/Refractory Multiple Myeloma. Blood 2020; 136: 26-27.

[73] Topp MS, Duell J, Zugmaier G et al. Anti-B-Cell Maturation Antigen BiTE Molecule AMG 420 Induces Responses in Multiple Myeloma. J Clin Oncol 2020; 38: 775-783.

[74] Lesokhin AM, Raje N, Gasparetto CJ et al. A Phase I, Open-Label Study to Evaluate the Safety, Pharmacokinetic, Pharmacodynamic, and Clinical Activity of PF-06863135, a B-Cell Maturation Antigen/CD3 Bispecific

Antibody, in Patients with Relapsed/ Refractory Advanced Multiple Myeloma. Blood 2018; 132: 3229-3229.

[75] Lesokhin AM, Levy MY, Dalovisio AP et al. Preliminary Safety, Efficacy, Pharmacokinetics, and Pharmacodynamics of Subcutaneously (SC) Administered PF-06863135, a B-Cell Maturation Antigen (BCMA)-CD3 Bispecific Antibody, in Patients with Relapsed/Refractory Multiple Myeloma (RRMM). Blood 2020; 136: 8-9.

[76] Parry RV, Chemnitz JM, Frauwirth KA et al. CTLA-4 and PD-1 receptors inhibit T-cell activation by distinct mechanisms. Mol Cell Biol 2005; 25: 9543-9553.

[77] Paiva B, Azpilikueta A, Puig N et al. PD-L1/PD-1 presence in the tumor microenvironment and activity of PD-1 blockade in multiple myeloma. Leukemia 2015; 29: 2110-2113.

[78] Chen D, Tang P, Liu L et al. Bone marrow-derived mesenchymal stem cells promote cell proliferation of multiple myeloma through inhibiting T cell immune responses via PD-1/PD-L1 pathway. Cell Cycle 2018; 17: 858-867.

[79] Mateos M-V, Orlowski RZ, Siegel DSD et al. Pembrolizumab in combination with lenalidomide and low-dose dexamethasone for relapsed/ refractory multiple myeloma (RRMM): Final efficacy and safety analysis. Journal of Clinical Oncology 2016; 34: 8010-8010.

[80] Mateos MV, Orlowski RZ, Ocio EM et al. Pembrolizumab combined with lenalidomide and low-dose dexamethasone for relapsed or refractory multiple myeloma: phase I KEYNOTE-023 study. Br J Haematol 2019; 186: e117-e121.

[81] Badros A, Hyjek E, Ma N et al. Pembrolizumab, pomalidomide, and low-dose dexamethasone for relapsed/ refractory multiple myeloma. Blood 2017; 130: 1189-1197.

[82] Mateos MV, Blacklock H, Schjesvold F et al. Pembrolizumab plus pomalidomide and dexamethasone for patients with relapsed or refractory multiple myeloma (KEYNOTE-183): a randomised, open-label, phase 3 trial. Lancet Haematol 2019; 6: e459-e469.

[83] Usmani SZ, Schjesvold F, Oriol A et al. Pembrolizumab plus lenalidomide and dexamethasone for patients with treatment-naive multiple myeloma (KEYNOTE-185): a randomised, open-label, phase 3 trial. Lancet Haematol 2019; 6: e448-e458.

Chapter 5

The Modern Age of Monoclonal Antibodies: The Revolution of Daratumumab

Gianfranco Lapietra, Francesca Fazio and Maria Teresa Petrucci

Abstract

CD38 is a transmembrane glycoprotein expressed on the surface of different cell lines with several functions (receptor, adhesion molecule, ectoenzyme). Based on its high expression in multiple myeloma cells, CD38 is one of the main molecules used in the target therapy age. Daratumumab is the first fully human monoclonal antibody tested in clinical trials, showing efficacy in relapsed/refractory multiple myeloma patients, especially in combination with immunomodulants and/or proteasome inhibitors. The synergic effect concerns multiple myeloma cells as well as the microenvironment (NK cells, macrophage, regulatory B/T cells and CD8+ effector cells). Therefore, the anti-multiple myeloma activity of Daratumumab greatly depends on the immune system: this is the reason why several ongoing clinical trial are testing its efficacy in the naïve patients, with a more effective immune system.

Keywords: daratumumab, monoclonal antibody, anti-CD38, multiple myeloma

1. Introduction: mechanism of action

Daratumumab is the first fully IgG_1K-human monoclonal antibody targeting CD38.CD38, also known as cyclic ADP ribose hydrolase, is a transmembrane glycoprotein expressed on the surface of hematopoietic and non-hematopoietic cell lines.

This protein plays different functions, both on the external and on the inner surface of cells. As a receptor, it takes part into the inflammatory response, stimulating the production of a great variety of cytokines through the interaction with CD31, on the surface of T cells. As enzyme, it is involved in the metabolism of nicotinamide adenine dinucleotide (NAD+), leading to the synthesis of cyclic ADP ribose (cADPR) which regulates cellular calcium trafficking [1].

In the context of bone niche, CD38 expression is very high on the surface of plasma cells. Pioneering studies have shown that this glycoprotein plays a key-role in the oncogenesis of multiple myeloma: increased intracellular levels of NAD+ seem to be associated with a less susceptibility to apoptosis [2] and the synthesis of cADPR favours the escape of tumour cells from the immune system [3]. In vitro, CD38 seems also to be associated with the formation of nanotubes that transfer mitochondria from the stromal cells to myeloma cells, boosting myeloma cell proliferation and survival [4].

IntechOpen

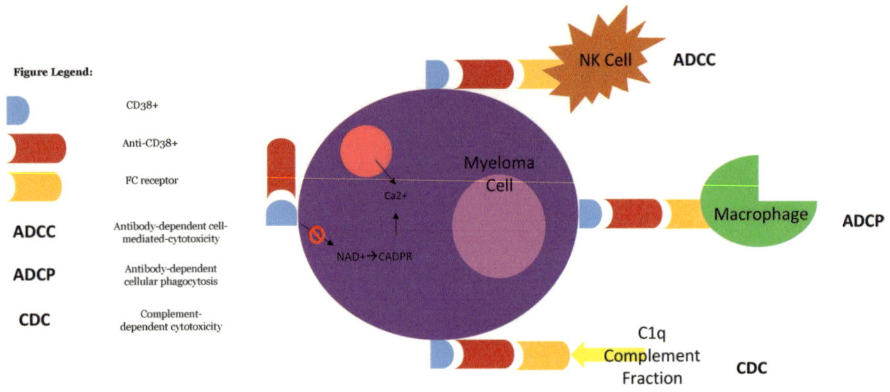

Figure 1.
Mechanism of action of daratumumab. Daratumumab binds CD38, killing myeloma cells via Fc-dependent immune effector mechanisms: CDC, ADCC and ADCP. Daratumumab also inhibits enzymatic activity of CD38, downregulating intracellular Ca^{2+} trafficking.

Daratumumab binds CD38, killing tumour cells via Fc-dependent immune effector mechanisms including complement-dependent cytotoxicity (CDC), antibody-dependent cell-mediated cytotoxicity (ADCC) and antibody-dependent cellular phagocytosis (ADCP) [5]. The complement activation seems to be the most effective mechanism used by Daratumumab [6]: the Fc tail of the drug binds the activating factor C1q leading both to ultimate activation of membrane attack complex and to deposition of C3b on the surface of multiple myeloma plasma cells. The activation of membrane attack complex causes osmotic lysis of cells while the deposition of complement factors attracts phagocytic cells. The recruitment of immune effector cells is also boosted by the release of circulating factors such as C3 and C5a (**Figure 1**).

The anti-tumour activity of Daratumumab does not depend only on the direct action on plasma cells but also on the interaction with other lymphoid and myeloid cells with a weak expression of CD38: NK cells, B and T regulatory cells and CD8+ effector cells. Krejcik et al. have demonstrated that bone marrow and peripheral blood from patients on treatment with Daratumumab present low levels of regulatory cells and high levels of NK and CD8+ effector cells. This monoclonal antibody may interfere with the immunosuppressive microenvironment in the multiple myeloma bone niche, in favour of major susceptibility for the plasma cells to the NK and CD8+ cells toxicity [7].

2. Pharmacokinetics

Daratumumab is usually administered at the dosage of 16 mg/kg weekly for 8 weeks then every 2 weeks for 16 weeks and every 4 weeks thereafter until progression of disease. The administration on a mg/kg basis is due to the observation that distribution and clearance of daratumumab depends on bodyweight. It seems to be not influenced by age, gender, race, mild renal and liver impairment. To our knowledge, the extra-liver metabolism of daratumumab is the reason for the absence of interactions with other drugs.

The efficacy and safety of this schedule have been demonstrated by two studies involving patients with relapsed/refractory multiple myeloma (RRMM) treated with the anti-CD38 monoclonal antibody as single agent: GEN501 and SIRIUS.

GEN501 was a phase I/II, open-label, multicenter study. In the dose-escalation part, sequential cohorts of patients received intravenous doses of daratumumab ranging from 0.005 to 24 mg/kg, administered over 6–8 h. In the dose-expansion study, in three of the enrolled cohorts, daratumumab was administered based on the findings from the previous part at 8 mg/kg weekly for 8 weeks, every 2 weeks for 16 weeks, and every 4 weeks until disease progression [8].

SIRIUS was a phase II study with two parts. In the first part, the patients were randomized to receive daratumumab 8 mg/kg every 4 weeks or 16 mg/kg weekly for 8 weeks, then every 2 weeks for 16 weeks and every 4 weeks thereafter. In the second part, all patients received daratumumab 16 mg/kg, according to the findings from the first part [9].

Intravenous administration of Daratumumab is associated with several side effects, included infusion-related reactions (see below). Therefore, this formulation requires a very slow infusion rate which may represent a disadvantage for the patient. Sever trials are evaluating the subcutaneous administration as an alternative. In the phase 1b PAVO study, the subcutaneous formulation of the monoclonal antibody was administered in patients with RRMM in combination with the recombinant human hyaluronidase PH20 enzyme (rHuPH20) to depolymerize hyaluronan in the subcutaneous space and increase the absorption rate [10]. This formulation at the dosage of 1800 mg was well tolerated and allowed to obtain similar concentrations and responses to the intravenous administration. Non-inferiority of subcutaneous daratumumab to intravenous formulation has been confirmed by preliminary results of the ongoing phase III trial COLUMBA [11]: enrolled patients with RRMM are randomized to receive either intravenous daratumumab 16 mg/kg or subcutaneous daratumumab 1800 mg. According to these studies, the approval of this formulation by the regulatory bodies is on the agenda.

3. Daratumumab in relapsed/refractory multiple myeloma

Approval of daratumumab by regulatory bodies was made possible thanks to clinical trials evaluating its use in RRMM. Patients with RRMM still represent the patients best benefitting from this monoclonal antibody, both as single agent and in combination with other agents (**Table 1a**).

3.1 Daratumumab in relapsed/refractory multiple myeloma as single agent

GEN501 and SIRIUS are the two main trials who led to approval of monotherapy with daratumumab. Both studies enrolled patients with RRMM: patients in GEN501 had relapsed after or were refractory to ≥2 prior lines of therapy, including inhibitors of proteasome (PIs), immunomodulatory drugs (IMiDs), chemotherapy and autologous stem cell transplantation (ASCT); patients in SIRIUS had relapsed after ≥3 lines of therapy, including a PI and a IMiDs or were double refractory to the most recently received PI and IMiDs. The primary endpoint of GEN501 was evaluation of safety while SIRIUS was designed to first evaluate overall response rate (ORR). Data regarding 148 patients from pooled analysis of the two trials confirmed how daratumumab, at the dosage of 16 mg/kg, is effective and safe in a population of heavily pretreated patients [12]. With a median number of 12 infusions, the ORR was 31.1%. At the time of the analysis, after a median follow-up of 20.7 months, the progression free survival (PFS) was 4 months, with a 12-month PFS rate of 22%. Stratifying the patients by the response according to International Myeloma Working Group, the PFS and the overall survival (OS) went out to be 15 months and not reached respectively for responders, 3 months and 18.5 months for patients with a stable disease or minimal response, 0.9 months and 3.7 months for non-responders. The median duration of response was 7.6 months and it deepened and improved in patients continuing daratumumab.

Trial	Phase	Therapy	Primary outcome
(a) RRMM			
GEN501	1/2	IV daratumumab single agent	evaluation of safety
SIRIUS	2	IV daratumumab single agent	ORR
PAVO	1B	SC daratumumab	Maximum ctrough N° of patients with AEs
COLUMBA	3	IV daratumumab *vs* SC daratumumab	ORR Maximum ctrough
NCT01615029	1 / 2	DARA-Rd	ORR
CASTOR	3	DARA-Vd *vs* Vd	PFS
POLLUX	3	DARA-Rd *vs* Rd	PFS
(b) NDMM			
ALCYONE	3	DARA-VMP *vs* VMP	PFS
MAIA	3	DARA-Rd *vs* DARA-Rd	PFS
CASSIOPEIA	3	DARA-VTd *vs* VTd	sCR after consolidation PFS
GRIFFIN	2	DARA-RVd *vs* RVd	sCR after consolidation
PERSEUS	3	DARA-RVd *vs* RVd	PFS

RRMM: Relapsed/Refractory Multiple Myeloma, IV: intravenous, SC: subcutaneous, Rd.: lenalidomide-dexamethasone, Vd: bortezomib-dexamethasone, ORR: Overall Response Rate, Maximum CTrough: Maximum Concentration Trough, AEs: Advese Events, PFS: Progression Free Survival, NDMM: Newly Diagnosed Multiple Myeloma, VMP: bortezomib-melphalan-dexamethasone, VTd: bortezomib-thalidomide-dexamethasone, RVd: lenalidomide-botrezomib-dexamethasone, sCR: stringent Complete Response.

Table 1.
Overview of main trials using Daratumumab in (a) RRMM, (b) NDMM.

3.1.1 Daratumumab in relapsed/refractory multiple myeloma in combination therapies: with IMiDs

Efficacy of daratumumab seems to be strengthened by other drugs used for multiple myeloma, given the synergic action on the immune system. As said before, the anti-CD38 may stimulate NK and T-cells, restoring "tumor suppressive immunological surveillance". Also IMiDs could increase the amount of regulatory cells in the bone niche, through inhibition of some transcriptional factors (Ikaros and Aialos) and the subsequent production of interleukin 2 [13]. Furthermore, some studies show that the main target of daratumumab is upregulated by action of IMiDs [14]. NCT01615029 was the first trial exploring the applicability of these laboratory observations, investigating efficacy of daratumumab in combination with lenalidomide and dexamethasone (Rd) [15]. It was a phase 1/2 study addressed to patients with relapsed multiple myeloma: phase 1 was a dose-escalation study in which the dose of 16 mg/kg for daratumumab was again determined; phase 2 was a dose-expansion study using the recommended dose of the first part. The three drugs were administered in cycle of 28 days: daratumumab was given according to the standard schedule, lenalidomide at 25 mg/day from days 1 to 21 of each cycle and dexamethasone at 40 mg/week. This combination revealed to be safe and very effective: the 18-months PFS rate was 72% and ORR was 81%, in this case too with an improvement of responses in time. To evaluate the advantage of adding daratumumab to a regimen with lenalidomide and dexamethasone, from 2014 to 2015, a phase III, randomized trial was carried out across Europe, Northern America and Asia [16]. The POLLUX trial enrolled 569 patients with multiple myeloma who had received one or more previous lines of therapy: 286 were assigned to the daratumumab group (daratumumab plus lenalidomide and dexamethasone) and 283 to the control group (lenalidomide and dexamethasone). Also in this trial, each cycle was of 28 days, with daratumumab administered according to the usual schedule, lenalidomide at 25 mg/day from days 1 to 21 of each cycle and dexamethasone at a dose of 40 mg weekly. At 12 months, the PFS rate was 83.2% in the daratumumab group *vs* 60.1% in the control group. In a sub analysis, this extension of PFS in the experimental group went out to be independent from the number of previous lines of therapy and from the previous exposure to lenalidomide, even if the paucity of refractory patients to IMiDs enrolled in this trial may represent a bias. After a follow-up of 13.5 months, progression disease or death occurred in 53 patients in the daratumumab group *vs* 116 patients in the control arm, with a hazard ratio of 0.37 in favour of the first group. Also in this case, an improvement of deepness of molecular response was observed with continuation of therapy with the monoclonal antibody and it translated in a longer survival. Indeed, 22.4% of patients in the experimental group had results below the threshold for minimal residual disease (MRD), compared to 4.6% in the control group. Neutropenia, diarrhea and infusional reactions were the main adverse events reported in the experimental arm with a higher incidence than in the control group but, in spite of that, the rate of grade 3 and grade 4 infections was not so different. In conclusion, POLLUX trial confirmed the efficacy and safety of adding daratumumab to a regimen with IMiDs and high-dose steroid. Furthermore, the excellent results below the threshold for minimal residual disease suggest that minimal residual disease negativity could represent a goal also for RRMM patients.

3.1.2 Daratumumab in relapsed/refractory multiple myeloma in combination therapies: with PIs

Some *in-vitro* studies have shown that not only IMiDs but also PIs interact with daratumumab in a synergic way, strengthening its effect. An assay performed by the Dutch group [14] evaluated the rate of lysis in samples of bone marrow mononuclear cells from 16 multiple myeloma patients incubated with medium containing either daratumumab, lenalidomide and bortezomib or just one drug. The rate of lysis went out to be higher in the samples with the addition of daratumumab, showing that not only lenalidomide but also bortezomib enhance the effect of this monoclonal antibody by sensitizing the cells to the antibody-mediated lysis. The "lysis effect" was even better in cells from patients who previously showed refractoriness to IMiDs or IPs, suggesting that immunomodulatory effects of daratumumab may restore host susceptibility to anti-myeloma agents. Based on a phase 1b trial in which daratumumab showed encouraging results in combination with PIs-based regimens in naive patients [17], a phase 3 trial randomized patients with relapsed and/or refractory multiple myeloma to a treatment with only bortezomib and dexamethasone or with the addition of daratumumab [18]. Of 498 patients, 251 were assigned to the daratumumab group and 247 to the control group. Each cycle had a duration of 21 days. Daratumumab was administered at the usual dosage of 16 mg/kg once per week during cycles 1 to 3, once every 3 weeks during cycles 4 to 8 and once every 4 weeks thereafter until toxicity or progression disease. Dexamethasone was given for a total dose of 160 mg per cycle and bortezomib was administered in the subcutaneous formulation at the dosage of 1.3 mg per square meter on days 1, 4, 8 and 11 of cycles 1 to 8. The 12-month rate of PFS was 60.7% in the experimental group and 26.9% in the control group. After a follow up of 7.4 months, progression disease or death occurred in 67 patients in the daratumumab group *vs* 122 in the control group. Given the results of the interim analysis, the trial was unblended earlier and patients in the control group with a progression disease were offered daratumumab monotherapy. This may represent a bias in the interpretation of all the long-term results. Nevertheless, this trial showed how daratumumab could give an advantage also in combination with PIs-based regimens. The recorded responses are deep and durable. The main adverse events reported in the daratumumab group were thrombocytopenia and infusion-related reactions but none of them led to a treatment discontinuation higher than in the control group.

3.1.3 Daratumumab in relapsed/refractory multiple myeloma in combination therapies: the experience from the Multiple Myeloma GIMEMA Lazio Group

Fazio et al. performed a multicentre retrospective analysis of patients with relapsed/refractory multiple myeloma treated with IMiDs or IPs-based regimens containing daratumumab in the hospitals of the GIMEMA (Gruppo Italiano Malattie Ematologiche dell'Adulto) network in the Italian region of Lazio [19]. Of 188 patients, sixty-five performed at least one cycle of therapy and were evaluable for hematologic response. The ORR was 81.97%; with four patients (6.56%) achieving a stringent complete response (sCR), 20 (32.79%) patients a complete response (CR), 5 (8.2%) patients a non-complete response (NCR), 13 (21.31%) patients a very good partial response (VGPR) and 8 (13.11%) patients a partial response (PR). After a median follow-up of 8.8 (range 0.23–22.3) months, 50 (42.37%) patients were alive maintaining response, eight (13.11%) patients presented a progression disease and one (1.64%) patients died. The overall survival and progression-free survival were 86.3% (95% CI, 79.2–94) and 70.8% (95% CI, 61.2–82), respectively. The most common grade 3 or 4 hematologic treatment-emergent adverse events (TAEs) included neutropenia, anemia and thrombocytopenia. The most common non-hematologic TAEs, of any grade, were infections, peripheral sensory neuropathy (7.6%) and fatigue (7.6%). Among the cases of infection, 17 (26%) patients presented pneumonia, eight (12%) patients FUO and five (7.7%) patients viral reactivation. Our preliminary results confirm data from POLLUX and CASTOR trial, suggesting that treatment with daratumumab in combination with lenalidomide or bortezomib plus dexamethasone is a highly effective and well-tolerated regimen to be considered for multiple myeloma patients after first relapse.

3.1.4 Daratumumab in relapsed/refractory multiple myeloma in combination therapies: with other novel agents

In the setting of heavily pretreated myeloma patients, daratumumab has shown good results also in association with novel drugs belonging to the last generations of IMiDs and IPs. Both combination of daratumumab with pomalidomide and dexamethasone and with carfilzomib and dexamethasone allowed to obtain deep and durable responses with a tolerable toxicity profile [20, 21]. Therefore, it seems reasonable to use daratumumab in combination with triplets or quadruplets in RRMM to obtain the best response.

3.2 Daratumumab in relapsed/refractory multiple myeloma in combination therapy: after or before allogenic hematopoietic cell-transplantation for young patients?

Despite improvements in the MM outcome and in the depth and response duration following subsequent lines of therapy, MM remains an incurable disease. It is reasonable to consider allogenic (allo) hematopoietic cell transplantation (HCT) as a treatment strategy for young patients with high-risk disease and an available donor. Allo-HCT is potentially effective by virtue of a graft-versus-myeloma (GvM) effect but currently, there is little available data regarding this treatment [22]. Given the action of daratumumab on the microenvironment, it could be used both to control the graft-versus-host disease and to improve the GvM effect. In the review by Nikolaenko et al., 34 patients treated with daratumumab after aploidentical HCT were evaluated [23]. The ORR after the treatment with the monoclonal antibody was 41%, only five cases of acute GVHD were reported and no cases of chronic GVHD, showing the efficacy of this strategy on a population of high-risk heavily pretreated patients. Based on this little data, we may speculate that the modification of microenvironment induced by daratumumab could be used to "plow the land" for the transplant. To our knowledge, none is known about the use of anti-CD38 as a bridge to the transplant. We recently reported the case of a young patients with relapsed myeloma after the standard induction therapy and a tandem ASCT who underwent 11 cycles of rescue therapy with daratumumab in combination with lenalidomide and dexamethasone, followed by haploidentical transplant. Thanks to this treatment, he achieved a partial response and is now on consolidation with Daratumumab-Rd regimen [24].

4. Daratumumab in untreated newly diagnosed multiple myeloma

More recently, the use of daratumumab has been also explored in the setting of newly diagnosed multiple myeloma (NDMM) patients, showing encouraging results both in the population of transplant eligible patients and in that of transplant ineligible patients. The first results about daratumumab in NDMM patients proceed from a phase 1b study evaluating tolerability and safety of this monoclonal antibody in combination with myeloma backbone regimens: bortezomib-dexamethasone (VD), bortezomib-thalidomide-dexamethasone (VTD), bortezomib-melphalan-dexamethasone (VMP), pomalidomide-dexamethasone (PD) [25]. NDMM patients were included in all the arms except the PD one: in the VD and VTD arms the patients were enrolled irrespective of the transplant eligibility, while all patients in the VMP arm were transplant ineligible. In all the four arms, daratumumab was well tolerated and safe (**Table 1b**).

4.1 Daratumumab in untreated newly diagnosed multiple myeloma: transplant ineligible patients

ALCYONE and MAIA are the two main trials which evaluated the efficacy of adding daratumumab in the standard treatment of untreated patients with multiple myeloma ineligible to transplant. ALCYONE enrolled 706 naive patients randomized to receive VMP alone or with daratumumab [26]. Each cycle had a duration of 42 days. In the control group, all the patients received up to nine cycles of subcutaneous bortezomib, administered at the dosage of 1.3 mg per square meter of body-surface area (twice weekly on weeks 1, 2, 4, and 5 of cycle 1 and once weekly on weeks 1, 2, 4, and 5 of cycles 2 through 9), oral melphalan (9 mg per square meter, once daily on days 1 through 4 of each cycle), and oral prednisone (60 mg per square meter, once daily on days 1 through 4 of each cycle). In the experimental group, intravenous daratumumab at the usual dose of 16 mg/kg was administered with oral or intravenous dexamethasone at a dose of 20 mg once weekly in cycle 1, every 3 weeks in cycles 2 through 9, and every 4 weeks thereafter until disease progression or toxicity. Dexamethasone at a dose of 20 mg was substituted for prednisone on day 1 of each cycle. At 12 months, the PFS was 86.7% in the daratumumab group *vs* 76.0% in the control group. At the clinical data cut-off, an event of disease progression or death had occurred in 88 (25.1%) patients in the daratumumab group *vs* 143 (40.2%) patients in the control group, with a hazard-ratio of 0.50 in favour of the first group. The superiority was even confirmed in the older patients, in those with a poor performance status and worse stage. It seemed to be also independent from impairment of renal and liver function which were quite frequent in the enrolled population. In spite of this general advantage given adding daratumumab, a prespecified subgroup analysis of progression-free survival showed that the D-VMP combination is not so effective in the overcome of the bad prognosis given by the high-risk cytogenetics (defined by t (4;14), t (14;16), del17p). The main adverse effect was represented by infections of the respiratory tract but they were not a cause of discontinuation of treatment. MAIA compared Rd. to daratumumab-Rd [27]. The trial enrolled 737 naïve patients: in cycles of 28 days, all of them received oral lenalidomide 25 mg on days 1 through 21 and oral dexamethasone 40 mg per week, until disease progression or toxicity. In the experimental group, daratumumab was added at a dose of 16 mg/kg once weekly during cycles 1 and 2, every 2 weeks during cycles 3 through 6, and every 4 weeks thereafter. At the median follow-up of 28 months, PFS was not reached in the daratumumab group and was 31.9 months in the control group. Disease progression or death occurred in 97 patients in the experimental group *vs* 143 in the control group, with a hazard-ratio of 0.56. Also in this trial, the benefit was maintained in older patients with worse performance status but not in the patients with high-risk cytogenetics. Pneumonia was recorded as the most frequent side effect in the experimental group but it did not influence the general outcome. Based on the exciting results of ALCYONE and MAIA, several ongoing trials throughout the world aim to evaluate the benefit of adding both subcutaneous and intravenous daratumumab to the different combinations of drugs used for the induction of multiple myeloma in naïve unfit patients (NCT03993912, NCT03742297, NCT03652064, NCT03217812, NCT04052880, NCT04009109, NCT03695744, NCT02918331). Some of these are designed to study possibility of combining the monoclonal antibody with the newest generations of IMiDs and IPs: NCT4009109 is a phase II trial with two arms based on induction with lenalidomide, ixazomib, daratumumab and dexamethasone; maintenance in arm 1 is with the only lenalidomide, in the arm 2 it is with lenalidomide, ixazomib and daratumumab. Ixazomib is a last-generation IPs which recently received the approval to be used in combination with lenalidomide and steroid in RRMM. The interim analysis of this phase II trial showed an overall response rate (ORR) of 70%, with good molecular response [28].

4.2 Daratumumab in untreated newly diagnosed multiple myeloma: transplant eligible patients

The excellent results achieved in the population of unfit NDMM patients led to evaluate the efficacy of daratumumab also in the population of NDMM transplant eligible patients. CASSIOPEIA trial is the first largest study going in this direction: it enrolled 1085 patients across Europe, randomly assigned to the control arm with the use of VTD triplet or to the experimental arm adding daratumumab [29]. All patients received up to four 28-day, pre-transplant induction cycles and two 28-day, post-transplant consolidation cycles of subcutaneous bortezomib (administered according to the usual schedule), oral thalidomide (100 mg daily in all cycles), and oral or intravenous dexamethasone. Daratumumab was administered intravenously at a dose of 16 mg/kg of bodyweight once weekly in induction cycles 1 and 2 and once every 2 weeks during induction cycles 3 and 4 and consolidation. At 100 days post-transplant, the rate of sCR was higher in the daratumumab group than in the control group (29% *vs* 20%) and this superiority was maintained in older patients, but not in patients with a higher stage disease and a higher risk cytogenetics. Also in this trial the main adverse events were represented by infections but none of them represented a cause of treatment discontinuation. Surprisingly, daratumumab went out to be associated with a reduction of the amount of collected stem cells CD34+ and the subsequent use of plerixafor, even if this aspect did not translate into a worse performance of the transplant. Recently, Voorhees et al. published the results of another study evaluating the use of daratumumab as first line in transplant eligible patients, the GRIFFIN trial [30]. In this phase II randomized trial, 207 enrolled patients received four 21-day induction cycles and two 21-day consolidation cycles of oral lenalidomide (25 mg daily on days 1–14), subcutaneous bortezomib (1.3 mg/m2 on days 1, 4, 8, and 11), and oral dexamethasone (VRD), followed by maintenance with lenalidomide until toxicity or progression disease. Patients in the experimental group received daratumumab (16 mg/kg) on days 1, 8, and 15 of cycles 1 through 4 and day 1 of consolidation cycles and of maintenance cycles. After the end of post-transplant consolidation, the primary end-point of sCR was achieved in 42 patients in the experimental group *vs* 31 patients in the control group. Also the secondary end-points of overall response rate and rate of VGPR or better resulted higher in the daratumumab group. These good results deepened over time. The observed benefit was maintained also in the older population but not again in patients with a higher disease stage and with high-risk cytogenetics. As usually observed, also in this trial the experimental arm recorded a high rate of not statistically significant infections. Several ongoing trials aim to evaluate the use of daratumumab as first-line in transplant eligible NDMM patients: among these, PERSEUS is a promising ongoing phase III trial evaluating efficacy of daratumumab plus VRD *vs* VRD in terms of PFS, utilizing subcutaneous daratumumab to minimize toxicity. There are also few ongoing trials evaluating induction with daratumumab irrespective of transplant eligibility and some of them are based on MRD-driven therapies (MASTER trial). The results of all these studies are awaited.

5. Daratumumab in other plasma cell neoplasms

Given the promising results in the treatment of multiple myeloma with daratumumab, its use is being investigating also in the treatment of other plasma cell neoplasms, especially immunoglobulin light chain (AL) amyloidosis and smouldering myeloma (SMM).

5.1 Daratumumab in amyloidosis

AL amyloidosis is due to the production of misfolded immunoglobulin light chain by an aberrant plasma-cells clone. This pathologic protein deposits in a variety of organs, usually heart and kidney, causing serious dysfunction. In spite of good results showed by treatment of this disease with PIs and IMiDs [31, 32], there is still a significant proportion of patients that do not respond to these agents. Based on a variety of reports showing safety and efficacy of daratumumab in patients with relapsed/refractory AL amyloidosis [33–36], some perspective trials have been recently conducted. NCT028441033 is a phase II study led at Boston Medical Center and aimed to evaluate safety and tolerability of daratumumab in a cohort of 25 participants with relapsed/refractory AL amyloidosis. The preliminary results were encouraging, with only infusion reactions being reported as main side effect [37]. The ORR is instead the primary outcome of a multi-center phase II study across France and Italy (NCT02816476): it enrolled 35 patients with AL amyloidosis not in VGPR or better after previous treatment. The preliminary results showed an ORR of 59% with 44% of patients achieving at least a VGPR [38]. These good results are confirmed by a report with the collaboration of our group [39]: 59 patients out of 72 with relapsed/refractory AL amyloidosis achieved a hematologic response after eight infusions of daratumumab, single agent or combined with bortezomib and lenalidomide, and the quality of this response improved with the continuation of therapy. The demonstration of the efficacy of daratumumab in the treatment of AL amyloidosis provided the rationale for exploring its use earlier in the disease course. Hossein Taghizadeh MA et al. presented the case of two patients with advanced cardiac involvement who achieved a normalization of light chain levels within one cycle of therapy with the anti-CD38, without any serious adverse events in spite of the cardiac dysfunction [40]. A phase III trial comparing cyclophosphamide, bortezomib and dexamethasone with or without daratumumab in the first-line treatment of AL amyloidosis has recently completed the enrolment and the results are awaited (NCT03201965).

5.2 Daratumumab in SMM

Smouldering myeloma is defined by a medullar infiltration of clonal plasmacells ≥10% in the absence of symptoms. According to the Mayo Clinic criteria, M-protein >2 g/dl, medullar infiltration ≥20% and free-light chain ratio > 20 define risk categories. Patients with one, two and three of these criteria are considered to be at low, intermediate and high risk with 5-year progression of 23% in the low risk, 47% in the intermediate risk and 82% in the high risk [41]. However, in spite of the important risk of transformation into symptomatic disease, current guidelines recommend "watch and wait" even in people with high and intermediate risk smouldering myeloma. Since the earlier intervention may delay progression, different studies are evaluating the use of new drugs in this subset of patients. Daratumumab could be the perfect drug, given the efficacy and the tolerability showed in other subsets. Based on the good results of the CENTAURUS trial, a phase II study for patients with intermediate and high risk smouldering multiple myeloma, randomly assigned, in a 1:1:1 ratio, to receive one of three different schedules of daratumumab [42], a phase III trial has been designed (NCT03301220). In this study, patients with high-risk smouldering myeloma are randomized either to receive subcutaneous daratumumab or to be just monitored. Daratumumab is administered according to the usual schedule, until 39 cycles or up to 36 months or until confirmed disease progression or unacceptable toxicity. This study recently completed the enrolment and the results are still awaited but all the most recent findings suggest that the anti-CD38 could be used with safety and efficacy also in smouldering myeloma.

6. The dark side of daratumumab: adverse events

All pivotal studies leading to approval of daratumumab for the treatment of relapsed-refractory or newly diagnosed multiple myeloma showed a slight major susceptibility to infections in the studied populations. This risk seems to be due to the neutropenia and to the impairment of cellular immunity which is a direct consequence of targeting CD38 [43]. In the study by Nahi et al., nine patients out of 23 treated with daratumumab had viral and/or bacterial complications, mainly involving the respiratory tract. In these patients, assessment of circulating lymphocytes indicated a selective depletion of NK cells and viral reactivation after Daratumumab treatment. This finding is in line with data emerging from all the trials using anti-CD38-based regimens and suggest the necessity of screening for cytomegalovirus, Epstein–Barr virus and viral hepatitis before starting the treatment, therefore an adequate antiviral and antibacterial prophylaxis in the treated population. In the consensus document by ESCMID Study Group for Infections in Compromised Hosts (ESGICH), based on the pooled analysis of the two trials GEN501 an SIRIUS, daratumumab is associated also with an increased risk of varicella-zoster virus (VZV) infections, especially in the presence of combination therapy with protease inhibitors and/or corticosteroids [44]. Anti-herpesvirus prophylaxis with (val)acyclovir should be administered to VZV-seropositive patients at least 1 week before starting daratumumab therapy and for at least 12 weeks after its discontinuation. The consensus document also recommends seasonal-influenza vaccination. In the review of the drug conducted under the EMA's accelerated assessment program for drugs that are of major interest for public health, also thrombocytopenia and anemia are reported as the most common side effects, besides neutropenia [45]. In this same report, half of all patients experienced infusion-related reactions, mainly occurring at the first infusion. These reactions usually presented with nasal congestion, cough, throat irritation, chills, vomiting and nausea. Serious adverse reactions with bronchospasm, dyspnea, laryngeal edema, pulmonary edema and hypoxia have been also reported but in a few cases. Based on this phenomenon, EMA gave indication to premedicate every infusion with antihistamines, antipyretics and corticosteroids. Furthermore, oral corticorsteroids should be taken by all patients on the first and second day after all infusions. Patients on therapy with Daratumumab may present with positive indirect and direct Coombs test, due to the CD38 expression also on the red blood cells. This interference could complicate the safe provision of blood products to people on treatment with this drug. Chapuy et al. demonstrated that this "laboratory side effect" might be solved by incubating red blood cells with dithiothreitol (DTT) or trypsin [46]. These reagents remove the CD38 on the surface of red blood cells, easing routine compatibility testing. Evaluation of disease response in patients with multiple myeloma on treatment with daratumumab could also be complicated by this antibody. Given its proteic nature (IgG1), the drug can be confused with the endogenous monoclonal component during the interpretation of serum immunofixation electrophoresis (IFE). McCudden et al. proposed a daratumumab-specific immunofixation electrophoresis reflex assay (DIRA) using a mouse anti-daratumumab antibody in order to discriminate between endogenous myeloma protein and daratumumab [47]. Both Castor and Pollux trials showed a slight increase of rates of secondary primary cancers in the experimental arms, within 6 months after the initiation of trials [16, 18]. Most of the cases were non-melanocytes related cutaneous tumours and occurred in patients already treated with IMiDs and alkylating agents. Further studies and longer follow-up are needed to clarify the potential carcinogenicity of Daratumumab. Another concern, regarding the use of daratumumab, is due to the expression of CD38 on the surface of CD34+ hematopoietic progenitor cells. This could theoretically translate into a delay in stem cells collection for eligible patients to ASCT on treatment with the monoclonal antibody. Xun Ma et al. conducted an assay in which specimens of mobilized peripheral blood CD34 + cells from myeloma patients were evaluated to determine percentage of CD38 expression and later incubated with daratumumab and complement-rich human serum. First, CD38 is minimally expressed on CD34+ cells, compared to the control cell lines used. Furthermore, CDC did not occur, showing that, in vitro, daratumumab is not toxic to mobilized CD34 + progenitor cells from myeloma patients [48].

7. Conclusions

Daratumumab has showed proven efficacy and tolerability both in patients with RRMM and with NDMM, as confirmed in all the studies conducted during the last years. A deep and durable response with easy-to-control side effects was obtained using this monoclonal antibody. The revolutionary power of this new drug could be also extended to patients with other plasma cell neoplasms, such as AL amyloidosis and SMM. Given the specific mechanisms of action of daratumumab targeting both clonal plasma-cells and bone-niche microenvironment, further studies are warranted to better understand the correct timing to introduce this monoclonal antibody in the context of a sequential therapy. On a side, the immune-mediated plasma-cell killing, induced by daratumumab in the early phase of treatment, acts as a debulking for the disease; on the other side, the restoration of the immune system may boost other metabolic effects of the monoclonal antibody, in a later phase of therapy, when the control of the disease is better [49]. Based on these hypothesis, the retreatment with daratumumab after a wash-out period may seem reasonable. Therefore, the anti-CD38 is a revolutionary weapon: understanding the best moment to use it in the battle against multiple myeloma is the great challenge of the future.

Conflict of interests

GL and FF have nothing to declare. MTP served as a consultant or on an advisory board for and received honoraria from Janssen-Cilag, Celgene, Bristol-Myers Squibb,Amgen, Takeda and Sanofi.

Author details

Gianfranco Lapietra, Francesca Fazio and Maria Teresa Petrucci*
Hematology, Department of Translational and Precision Medicine,
Sapienza University, Rome, Italy

*Address all correspondence to: petrucci@bce.uniroma1.it

References

[1] Morandi F, Horenstein AL, Costa F et al. CD38: a target for immunotherapeutic approaches in multiple myeloma. Front Immunol. 2018; 9: 2722.

[2] Cagnetta A, Cea M, Calimeri T, et al. Intracellular NAD^+ depletion enhances bortezomib-induced anti-myeloma activity. Blood. 2013; 122(7):1243-1255.

[3] Chillemi A, Quarona V, Antonioli L, et al. Roles and Modalities of Ectonucleotidases in Remodeling the Multiple Myeloma Niche. Front Immunol. 2017; 8:305.

[4] Marlein CR, Piddock RE, Mistry JJ, et al. CD38-Driven Mitochondrial Trafficking Promotes Bioenergetic Plasticity in Multiple Myeloma. Cancer Res. 2019 May 1;79(9):2285-2297.

[5] van de Donk NWCJ, Usmani SZ. CD38 Antibodies in Multiple Myeloma: Mechanisms of Action and Modes of Resistance. Front Immunol. 2018 Sep 20; 9:2134.

[6] van de Donk NW, Janmaat ML, Mutis T, et al. Monoclonal antibodies targeting CD38 in hematological malignancies and beyond. Immunol Rev. 2016; 270:95-112.

[7] Krejcik J, Casneuf T, Nijhof IS, et al. Daratumumab depletes CD38+ immune regulatory cells, promotes T-cell expansion, and skews T-cell repertoire in multiple myeloma. Blood. 2016;128 (3):384-394.

[8] Lokhorst HM, Plesner T, Laubach JP, et al. Targeting CD38 with daratumumab monotherapy in multiple myeloma. N Engl J Med. 2015;373:1207-1219.

[9] Lonial S, Weiss B, Usmani S, et al. Daratumumab monotherapy in patients with treatment-refractory multiple myeloma (SIRIUS): an open-label, randomised, phase 2 trial. Lancet. 2016;387:1551-1560.

[10] Usmani SZ, Nahi H, Mateos MV, et al. Subcutaneous delivery of daratumumab in relapsed or refractory multiple myeloma. Blood. 2019;134(8):668-677.

[11] Mateos MV, Nahi H, Legiec W, et al. Subcutaneous versus intravenous daratumumab in patients with relapsed or refractory multiple myeloma (COLUMBA): a multicentre, open-label, non-inferiority, randomised, phase 3 trial. Lancet Haematol. 2020 May;7(5):e370-e380.

[12] Usmani SZ, Weiss BM, Plensrer T, et al. Clinical efficacy of daratumumab monotherapy in patients with heavily pretreated relapsed or refractory multiple myeloma. Blood. 2016;128(1):37-44.

[13] Gandhi AK, Kang J, Havens CG, et al. Immunomodulatory agents lenalidomide and pomalidomide co-stimulate T cells by inducing degradation of T cell repressors Ikaros and Aiaolos via modulation of the E3 ubiquitin ligase complex CRL4 (CRBN). Br J Haematol. 2014;164(6):811-821.

[14] van der Veer MS, de Weers M, van Kessel B, et al. The therapeutic human CD38 antibody daratumumab improves the anti-myeloma effect of newly emerging multi-drug therapies. Blood Cancer J. 2011; 1(10):e41.

[15] Plesner T, Arkenau H-T, Gimsing P, et al. Phase ½ study of daratumumab, lenalidomide, and dexamethasone for relapsed multiple myeloma. Blood. 2016; 128(14).1821-1828.

[16] Dimopoulos MA, Oriol A, Nahi H, et al. Daratumumab, lenalidomide, and

dexamethasone for multiple myeloma. N Engl J Med. 2016;375(14):1319-31.

[17] Chari A, Lonial S, Suvannasankha A, et al. Open-label, multicenter, phase 1b study of daratumumab in combination with pomalidomide and dexamethasone in patients with at least two lines of priori therapy and relapsed or relapsed and refractory multiple myeloma (MM). Presented at the American Society of Hematology 56th Annual Meeting and Exposition, San Francisco, December 6-9, 2015.

[18] Palumbo A, Chanan-Khan A, Weisel K, et al. Daratumumab, bortezomib, and dexamethasone for multiple myeloma. N Engl J Med. 2016;375(8):754-66.

[19] Fazio F, Sfara G, Vozella F, et al. Therapy regimens including daratumumab for relapsed/refractory multiple myeloma patients: report from the Multiple Myeloma GIMEMA Lazio Group. Presented at the European Hematology Association 25th Congress, Frankfurt, June 11-14, 2020.

[20] Chari A, Suvannasankha A, Fay JW, et al. Daratumumab plus pomalidomide and dexamethasone in relapsed and/ or refractory multiple myeloma. Blood. 2017 Aug 24;130(8):974-981.

[21] Chari A, Martinez-Lopez J, Mateos MV, et al. Daratumumab plus carfilzomib and dexamethasone in patients with relapsed or refractory multiple myeloma. Blood. 2019 Aug 1;134(5):421-431.

[22] Donato ML, Siegel DS, Vesole DH et al. The graft-versus-host disease but not acute graft-versus-host disease prolongs survival in patients with multiple myeloma receiving allogenic transplantation. Biol Blood Marrow Transplant 2014;20:1211-6.

[23] Nikolaenko L, Chabra S, Biran N, et al. Graft-Versus-Host Disease in Multiple Myeloma Patients Treated With Daratumumab After Allogeneic Transplantation. Clin Lymphoma Myeloma Leuk 2020 Jun;20(6):407-414.

[24] Fazio F, Quattrocchi L, Fiori L, et al. Daratumumab before and after haploidentical stem cell transplantation in relapsed/refractory multiple myeloma: is the right strategy to overcome microenvironment impact in multiple myeloma? J Clin Trials Res. In press.

[25] Moreau P, Mateos MV, Bladé J, et al. An open-label, multicenter, phase 1b study of daratumumab in combination with backbone regimens in patients with multiple myeloma. Blood. 2014;124:176.

[26] Mateos MV, imopoulos MA, Cavo M, et al. Daratumumab plus bortezomib, melphalan, and prednisone for untreated myeloma. N Engl J Med. 2018;378:518-528.

[27] Facon T, Kumar S, Plesner T, et al. Daratumumab plus lenalidomide and dexamethasone for untreated myeloma. N Engl J Med. 2019;380:2014-2115.

[28] Stege CAM, Nasserinejad K, Levin MD, et al. Efficacy and tolerability of ixazomib, daratumumab and low dose dexamethasone (IDd) in unfit and frail newly diagnosed multiple myeloma (NDMM) patients; first interim safety analysis of the phase II HOVON 143 study. Blood. 2018;132(Suppl. 1):596.

[29] Moreau P, Attal M, Hulin C, et al. Bortezomib, thalidomide, and dexamethasone with or without daratumumab before and after autologous stem-cell transplantation for newly diagnosed multiple myeloma (CASSIOPEIA): a randomised, open-label, phase 3 study. Lancet. 2019;394:29-38.

[30] Voorhees PM, Kaufman JL, Laubach J, et al. Daratumumab, lenalidomide, bortezomib, and dexamethasone for

transplant-eligible newly diagnosed multiple myeloma: the GRIFFIN trial. Blood. 2020;136(8):936-945.

[31] Palladini G, Sachchithanantham S, Milani P, et al. A European collaborative study of cyclophosphamide, bortezomib, and dexamethasone in upfront treatment of systemic AL amyloidosis. Blood. 2015; 126(5):612-5

[32] Cibeira MT, Oriol A, Lahuerta JJ, et al. A phase II trial of lenalidomide, dexamethasone and cyclophosphamide for newly diagnosed patients with systemic immunoglobulin light chain amyloidosis. Br J Haematol. 2015; 170(6):804-13

[33] Sanchez L, Wang Y, Siegel DS, et al. Daratumumab: a first-in-class CD38 monoclonal antibody for the treatment of multiple myeloma. J Hematol Oncol. 2016; 9(1): 51.

[34] Sher T, Fenton B, Akthar A, et al. Firs report of safety and efficacy of daratumumab in 2 cases of advanced immunoglobulin light chain amyloidosis. Blood. 2016; 128(15): 1987-9.

[35] Kimmich C, Schonland SO, Muller-Tidow C, et al. Daratumumab monotherapy in forty-eight heavily pretreated patients with advanced systemic light-chain amyloidosis. The XVIth International Symposium on Amyloidosis; March 26-29; Kumamoto, Japan 2018.

[36] Abeykoon JP, Zanwar S, Kumar S, et al. Daratumumab-based therapies in patients with AL amyloidosis. The XVIth International Symposium on Amyloidosis; March 26-29; Kumamoto, Japan 2018.

[37] Sanchorawala V, Sarosiek S, Sloan JM, et al. Safety and tolerability of daratumumab in patients with relapsed light chain (AL) amyloidosis: preliminary results of a phase II study. American Society of Hematology 59th Annual Meeting & Exposition; December 9-12; Atlanta, 2017.

[38] Roussel M, Stoppa A-M, Perrot A, et al. A prospective phase II of daratumumab in previously-treated systemic light-chain (AL) amyloidosis. Blood. 2017; 130 508.

[39] Milani P, Fazio F, Basset M,et al. High rate of profound clonal and renal responses with daratumumab treatment in heavily pre-treated patients with light chain (AL) amyloidosis and high bone marrow plasma cell infiltrate. Am J Hematol. 2020 Aug;95(8):900-905.

[40] Hossein Taghizadeh MA, Reiter T, Duca F, et al. Daratumumab- a safe first-line treatment of cardiac AL amyloidosis in heavily compromised patients. The XVIth International Symposium on Amyloiodosis March 26-29; Kumamoto, Japan 2018.

[41] Lakshan A, Rajkumar SV, Buadi FK, et al. Risk stratification of smoldering multiple myeloma incorporating revised IMWG diagnostic criteria. Blood Cancer J. 2018; 8:59.

[42] Landgren CO, Chari A, Cohen YC, et al. Daratumumab monotherapy for patients with intermediate-risk or high-risk smoldering multiple myeloma: a randomized, open-label, multicentre, phase 2 study (CENTAURUS). Leukemia. 2020; 34:1840-1852.

[43] Nahi H, Chrobok M, Gran C, et al. Infectious complications and NK cell depletion following daratumumab treatment of Multiple Myeloma. PLoS One. 2019;14(2):e0211927.

[44] Drgona L, Gudiol C, Lanini S, et al. ESCMID Study Group for Infections in Compromised Hosts (ESGICH) Consensus Document on the safety of targeted and biological therapies: an infectious diseases perspective (Agents targeting lymphoid

or myeloid cells surface antigens [II]: CD22, CD30, CD33, CD38, CD40, SLAMF-7 and CCR4). Clin Microbiol Infect. 2018 Jun;24 Suppl 2:S83-S94.

[45] Tzogani K, Penninga E, Christiansen MLS, et al. EMA Review of Daratumumab for the Treatment of Adult Patients with Multiple Myeloma. The Oncologist. 2018; 23:594-602.

[46] Chapuy CI, Nicholson RT, Aguad MD, et al. Resolving the daratumumab interference with blood compatibility testing. Transfusion. 2015; 55:1545-54.

[47] McCudden C, Axel AE, Slaets D, et al. Monitoring multiple myeloma patients treated with daratumumab: teasing out monoclonal antibody interference. Clin Chem Lab Med 2016; 54:1095-104.

[48] Ma X, Wong SW, Zhou P, et al. Daratumumab binds to mobilized CD34+ cells of myeloma patients in vitro without cytotoxicity or impaired progenitor cell growth. Exp Hematol Oncol. 2018;7:27.

[49] Plesner T, van de Donk N, Richardson PG. Controversy in the Use of CD38 Antibody for Treatment of Myeloma: Is High CD38 Expression Good or Bad? Cells. 2020 Feb 6;9(2):378.

Chapter 6

Pleural Effusion Secondary to Multiple Myeloma: Is Daratumumab an Effective Treatment? A Case Report

Giulia Palazzo, Lara Aprile, Giacomo Cecere, Vito Pier Gagliardi, Alessandro Maggi, Antonella Prudenzano and Patrizio Mazza

Abstract

Extramedullary (EM) plasmacytoma disease is an aggressive presentation at diagnosis and relapse for multiple myeloma (MM) patients. EM plasmacytoma is divided into two groups: the first group comprises tumors that extend directly from osteolytic bone lesions, while the second results from plasmacytoma infiltration into soft tissues, with no relation to the bone. Despite new therapies and monoclonal antibodies, the survival for patients with EM plasmacytoma is poor. The involvement of pleural effusion is uncommon in multiple myeloma.

Keywords: daratumumab, pleural effusion, extramedullary plasmacytoma, multiple myeloma, CD 38, PET/TC

1. Introduction

Solitary plasmacytoma (SP) is an infrequent form of plasma cell neoplasm according to literature data, accounting for between 5 and 10% of all plasma cell neoplasms.

It is characterized by the presence of neoplastic monoclonal plasma cells that do not have systemic distribution but gather in limited locations even if there is no systemic proliferative plasma cell disease.

We can divide it into two groups: solitary bone plasmacytoma (SBP) and extra medullary plasmacytoma (EMP).

When the localization is prevalent in the bones of the axial skeleton, skull type, vertebrae, etc., we speak of solitary plasmacytoma of the bone (SBP), while EMP, as a localization, is frequent in the nasal cavities and in the nasopharynx.

The mean age of patients with SBP or EMP, with a male–female ratio of SP 2:1, is 55 years.

With advancing age, the incidence rate increases exponentially while maintaining a lower incidence compared to multiple myeloma (MM).

In the black population, the impact of the SP is about 30% higher than that in the white population [1].

A better definition of the tumor mass can be obtained with the fluorodeoxyglucose-positron emission tomography (FDG-PET) or positron emission tomography-computed tomography (PET-CT) [2] that allows direct visualization of the tumor burden; combining the morphological images of the CT scan with a particular molecular process (depending on the radiopharmaceutical injected such as a glucose analogue, which is the most widely used) allows to evaluate the response to treatment and the prognosis of different cancers.

The limit of the skeletal X-ray investigation of the whole body (WBXR) is represented by showing only osteolysis related to the presence of MM cells, while the FDG-PET allows to view the tumor load.

Obviously, this investigation is not without limitations; one of which is the false - negative or false-positive result, which is possible if inflammatory or infectious processes are in progress or if subcentimetric lesions cannot be detected by FDG-PET.

Aid is provided by the combined CT component, which provides higher resolution bone images than those obtained with normal radiography.

Through a direct anatomical correlation of FDG uptake foci.

The systematic review reported by Van Lammeren-Venema et al. [3] also compared FDG-PET and FDG-PET/CT with WBXR and CT.

The detection rate of FDG-PET/CT, compared with WBXR, ranged from 1.27 to 1.45; specificity was low (29–50%) and sensitivity ranged from 67 to 100% when using WBXR as a reference test. Regelink et al. mentioned that FDG-PET underestimates rib lesions, as they could be detected by low-dose CT integrated into PET.

A limitation, to date not resolved, is the detection of cranial lesions that FDG-PET/CT does not detect due to the high absorption of FDG in the brain, while the identification of extramedullary disease was satisfactory with FDG-PET; this has been reported consistently in studies comparing FDG-PET/CT with WBXR.

In addition to FDG that is specific to glucose metabolism, other PET radiopharmaceuticals have been developed to visualize various biological processes; among these, we can mention 18F fluoride being reevaluated for skeletal imaging and the 11C-methionine amino acid analogue and 11C-choline, an analogue precursor of phosphatidylcholine, one of the main constituents of membrane lipids, which to date have only been evaluated in small series of patients with MM.

Multiple myeloma [4] is a clonal malignant plasma cell neoplasm that despite the development of new therapies that have improved the depth and duration of responses as well as survival, to date, remains incurable in most cases for many patients.

Understanding the biology of disease, technological advances, such as next-generation sequencing techniques, have shown that the disease is genetically extremely heterogeneous, and this has allowed us to stratify patients, based on risk, into different disease groups. This can significantly translate into the choice of therapy and clinical results.

Simultaneously with these new acquisitions, the therapeutic scenario has been completely revolutionized by the discovery of new therapeutic agents, including immunomodulatory drugs (IMiDs) such as lenalidomide and pomalidomide; proteasome inhibitors (PIs) including bortezomib, carfilzomib and ixazomib; monoclonal antibodies (MAbs) including daratumumab and elotuzumab; and histone deacetylase inhibitors such as panobinostat, which have helped improve the overall survival of patients with this disease.

The use of many new therapeutic agents, in addition to increasing therapeutic choices, has also changed our therapeutic reference models; in fact, over the years, the treatment of patients with this pathology has mainly been based on high-dose radiation, but today, in consideration of the new drugs available to us, studies are needed to evaluate their use and benefit also in this category of high-risk patients.

2. Case introduction

A 58-year-old woman was diagnosed asymptomatic Multiple Myeloma Ig G K, stage II (International staging system - ISS).

She first presented in March 2018 because about 15 days before she was admitted to the nephrology department for acute renal failure, macrohematuria, hydronephrosis, and renal colic.

For confirmation during hospitalization, the laboratory tests of the monoclonal component was sent to our clinic.

Physical examination was negative.

Blood chemistry tests revealed that protein electrophoresis showed a monoclonal spike (M spike) 1 g/dl: IgG tests 1000 mg/dl, IgM 34 mg/dl, IgA 44 mg/dl, serum kappa light chains 294 mg/dl, serum lambda light chains 24 mg/dl, urine kappa light chains 187 mg/L, urine lambda light chains <4.7 mg/dl, FLC ratio 58, beta 2 microglobulin: 4.3 mg/L, Hb 13 g/dl, normal creatinine and calcium, proteinuria 0.8 g/24 h, and microalbuminuria 68 mg/L.

At the evaluation of the bone biopsy, plasma cell clonality was equal to 10–40%. At the phenotypic analysis and morphological examination, plasma cell infiltrate was equal to 24% (**Table 1**).

The karyotype analysis was 46 XX normal karyotype, and the FISH study showed TP53 in 35% of the nuclei analyzed.

Whole-body MRI showed no bone lesions, and the total body CT was negative.

Therefore, we asked the patient to visit the clinic for periodic checks.

After one year from diagnosis, in May 2019, she reported back pain for which blood tests and instrumental tests TB CT and MRI were performed.

The total body CT showed the following: "In a context of widespread reduction in calcium content, suspicious osteostructural alterations due to secondary disease localization of the skeletal segments included in the study volume are not appreciated. Apex cuneiform deformation of the anterior trunk of D12, widespread spondyloarthrosis manifestations. No focal tomodensitometric alterations of current pathological significance affecting the lung parenchyma bilaterally. Non-ilo-mediastinal and laterocervical lymphadenomegaly. Non-pleural-pericardial effusion. No gross changes affecting the abdominal parenchymatous organs, distended bladder with regular walls, no adenomegaly at the level of the main abdominal-pelvic lymph node stations, no free abdominal fluid."

Unlike the CT, the MRI of the abdomen showed the following: "collapse of D12 and pathological tissue with a paravertebral site with abdominal tissue formation that concentrically englobes the aorta and pleural effusion."

The MRI of dorsal and lumbar spine showed the following: "at the level of the interbody space D11–D12, presence of posterior median disc protrusion, at the level of the interbody space D12–L1, presence of protrusion of the annulus fibrosus with posterior median expression."

The spinal cord presents regular morphology and no pathological signal.

Immunophenotypic study in flow cytometry
Method used direct immunofluorescence
Antigens studied: CD19, CD38, CD 138, CD 56, CD 45
Result
Clonal myeloma plasma cells: CD 138+ CD 38++ CD19-CD56+ bright CD 45 neg = 24%

Table 1.
Phenotypic analysis of bone biopsy.

At the level of the interbody space L3-L4 and L5-S1, there was the presence of disc protrusion.

The body of D12 appears crushed and deformed into a wedge; the vertebral body itself exhibits a hypointense signal in the images in T1 as from the presence of spongiosa edema in vertebral distress, probably of a recently established post traumatic type; also, at the dorsal level, it is possible to document the presence of a sleeve that seems to envelop the vertebral structures, in the front and in the antero-lateral position bilaterally, and that extends from D12 to D5.

From the blood tests, the following data were gathered: lipase increase 995 U/L, monoclonal component: 2.6 gr/dl, creatinine 1 mg/dl, calcium 9.8 mg/dl, LDH 172 U/l, HB 12.49 g/dl, protein in the urine: 1, 4 g/24/h, urine kappa light chains 604 mg/L, beta 2 microglobulin 5.2 mg/dl, creatinine clearance 68 mm/h, serum K light chains 570 mg/dl, creatinine clearance 63 ml/min, microalbuminuria 98 mg/L, immunoglobulins IgG 1950 mg/dl, IgA immunoglobulins 20 mg/dL, IgM immunoglobulins 22 mg/dL.

The radiotherapy evaluation did not indicate treatment and she was treated with VTD (bortezomib 1.3 mg/m2 days 1, 4, 8, 11, thalidomide 100 mg/day, and dexamethasone 40 mg days 1, 4, 8, 11) for six cycles, obtaining only temporary biochemical partial response but extramedullary progression with increased pleural effusion.

The total body PET/CT that was performed (3.12.19) highlighted the following: "presence of a very large area of net and inhomogeneous pathological hyperaccumulation of radio glucose coinciding with dense tissue on the co-registration CT, which is extended, in front of the rachis, from the first dorsal metamers (D3/D4) to the upper limiting of the soma of L5, displacing and, at times, partially incorporating the posterior mediastinal structures (esophagus) along its course, and, more completely, the large thoraco-abdominal vessels up to the aorto-iliac "carrefour," with SUV max up to 9.7."

A circumscribed and apparently more isolated area of pathological hyperaccumulation is observed at the height of the right lung apex, in the paravertebral, at the level of D2.

Isolated pathological hyperaccumulations of radioglucose are found in the anterior mediastinum, coinciding with pleuro-pericardial pseudonodulation, at the height of the posterior aspect of the xiphoid, in the right parasternal in the context of the chest wall, in the form of two circumscribed areas of which the most voluminous with standardized uptake value max up to 7.0 and the other smaller max up to 5.7.

On an ancillary basis, the coregistration CT images include extensive pleural effusion on the right and relatively more modest on the left (**Table 2**).

We also decided to perform the phenotypic analysis on peripheral blood that showed plasma cell equal to 1.6%* (**Table 3**).

She repeated bone marrow biopsy that showed plasma cell infiltration on morphological examination equal to 70%, while the phenotypic analysis on bone marrow blood showed plasma cell CD138+ CD38++ CD19- CD56+ bright CD45 low with clonal kappa restriction of intracytoplasmic = 13%* (**Table 4**).

Therefore, we decided to subject the patient to therapy with cyclophosphamide (1.5 gr/die, day 1 and day 3) for debulking plus evacuative thoracentesis; unfortunately, we did not perform phenotypic study of the pleural fluid, and subsequently, we started therapy with daratumumab, lenalidomide, and dexamethasone (daratumumab was initiated at the standard dose of 16 mg/kg for week IV for 4 infusions plus lenalidomide 25 mg daily for 21 of 28 days, and dexamethasone 40 mg on week (Dara Rd).

The treatment was well tolerated and no pulmonary or hematological adverse events occurred.

DOI: http://dx.doi.org/10.5772/intechopen.95659

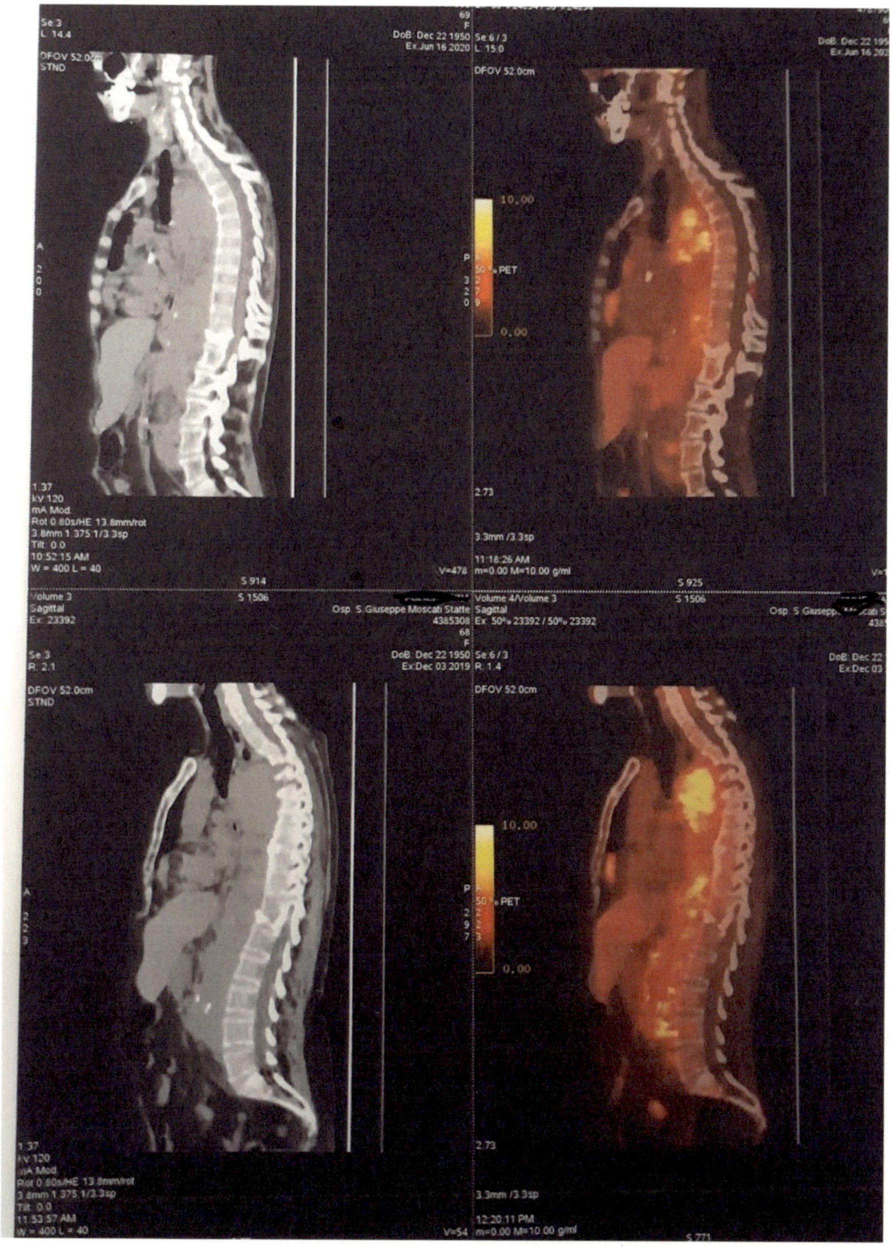

Table 2.
Image of PET.

Immunophenotypic study in flow cytometry
Method used direct immuno-fluorescence
Antigens studied: CD19, CD 20, CD 138, CD38, CD 56, CD 45, intracytoplasmatic chains kappa and lambda
Result
Mature lymphocytes = 8,6%
Clonal myeloma plasma cells: CD 138+ CD 38++CD19-CD56+ bright, CD 45 low with kappa clonal restriction = 1.6%

Table 3.
Phenotypic analysis on peripheral blood.

Immunophenotypic study in flow cytometry
Method used direct immunofluorescence
Antigens studied: CD19, CD 138, CD38, CD 56, chains kappa and lambda
Result
Mature lymphocytes = 20%
Clonal myeloma plasma cells: CD 138+ CD 38++CD19-CD56+ bright, CD 45 low with kappa clonal restriction = 13%

Table 4.
Phenotypic analysis on bone marrow blood.

Immunophenotypic study in flow cytometry
Method used direct immunofluorescence
Antigens studied: CD3, CD3/4, CD 3/CD8, CD19, CD16–56, CD117, CD 138, CD38, CD45, intracytoplasmatic chains kappa and lambda
Result
Mature lymphocytes = 60%
Clonal myeloma plasma cells: CD 138+ CD 38-, CD56+, CD 45 + heterogeneous, cy kappa + = 10%

Table 5.
Phenotypic analysis of pleural effusion.

Immunophenotypic study in flow cytometry
Method used direct immunofluorescence
Antigens studied: CD 19, CD 56, CD 138, CD38, CD45, cyVS38c.
RESULT
Mature lymphocytes = 40%
Clonal myeloma plasma cells: CD 138+ CD 38-*, CD56 + bright, cyvs38c+, CD 19- = 7.5%
*Therapy with Daratumumab

Table 6.
Phenotypic analysis of pleural effusion.

After one cycle of Dara Rd. therapy, for new reappearance of pleural effusion, the patient underwent thoracentesis, this time by performing the phenotypic analysis (**Table 5**).

While the plasma cells are absent for the reevaluation of the phenotypic study on peripheral blood, we continued the treatment until the fourth cycle.

After four cycles of therapy, we repeated PET/CT that was unfortunately compatible with persistence of disease.

The PET/CT showed persistence of a large area of hyperaccumulation of the tracer in coincidence of pathological tissue from D3 to L5 that incorporates the posterior mediastinal structures in its course.

Persistence of pathological accumulation in the anterior mediastinum, in the pleuro-pericardial region in increase compared to the previous examination, extending from the xiphoid to the anterior costophrenic recess, area of hyperaccumulation in the right parasternal and at the level of the mediastinal pleura close to the ascending aorta.

Despite the progression of disease, the CD38 negativity remained to the phenotypic reevaluation of the pleural fluid (**Table 6**).

3. Discussion

CD38 [5] is a transmembrane glycoprotein that is highly expressed on multiple myeloma cells and on normal lymphoid and myeloid cells albeit at low levels.

The mechanism of action is that of an ectoenzyme involved in the regulation of the intracytoplasmic concentration of calcium and of the catabolism of extracellular nucleotides.

The anti-CD38 fully human IgG1-k monoclonal antibody, daratumumab, carries out its cytotoxic effect through a series of mechanisms following binding to CD38, including antibody-dependent cell-mediated cytotoxicity (ADCC), complement-dependent cytotoxicity (CDC), antibody-dependent cell-mediated phagocytosis (ADCP), and direct induction of apoptosis, which are its main mechanisms of action.

Another effect of daratumumab recently described is its immunomodulatory action.

A phase I/II dose escalation study in 104 patients with relapsed or refractory multiple myeloma evaluated the safety of daratumumab.

The most common adverse events were grade 3 or 4 pneumonia and thrombocytopenia.

Two phase [5] III studies are evaluating patients with relapsed or refractory disease; one of these studies is comparing daratumumab plus bortezomib and dexamethasone versus bortezomib and dexamethasone and the other is comparing daratumumab plus lenalidomide and dexamethasone versus lenalidomide and dexamethasone.

Pending the final results of these studies, however, we want to underline how the CASTOR study (Velcade/dex vs. Dara/Velcade/dex) was interrupted early because at an interim analysis the study reached its final point with a ratio of very impressive risk of 0.39 in favor of the daratumumab arm. The POLLUX study (Rev/dex vs. Dara/Rev/dex) also showed similarly impressive results with a hazard ratio of 0.37 in favor of the Dara arm. Two further phase III studies are ongoing in patients with previously untreated multiple myeloma; one is comparing daratumumab plus bortezomib, melphalan, and prednisone with bortezomib, melphalan, and prednisone), and the other is evaluating daratumumab plus lenalidomide and dexamethasone with lenalidomide and dexamethasone.

We wanted to report this clinical case only to hypothesize a possible role of daratumumab in the treatment of extramedullary recurrences and above all its possible overcoming of the pleural barrier.

The selection of resistant clones is known in the course of myeloma recurrence, but the negativity/masking of CD 38 in the pleural fluid could demonstrate the overcoming of the pleural barrier by daratumumab.

Obviously we have no previous data, but the phenotypic analysis of the marrow and peripheral blood is the same for the other antigens evaluated.

Most likely, we should have performed a PET/CT at the onset of staging for a better evaluation of any extramedullary localization and perhaps choose different or more aggressive therapeutic treatments.

Molecular biology studies certainly in the near future will help us better understand which forms are most at risk and perhaps will guide us better in therapeutic choices.

But to date, the treatment of extramedullary plasmacytoma remains a therapeutic challenge even in the era of new drugs.

4. Conclusion

Despite significant progress in the treatment of multiple myeloma, the disease remains incurable in a vast majority of patients.

The approval of promising new agents will undoubtedly improve outcomes for myeloma patients.

Daratumumab is a monoclonal antibody that is now approved for treatment of multiple myeloma patients and has shown significant response in the real-world setting.

Our case illustrates the potential to overcome the pleural membrane and therefore a possible role also in the treatment of extramedullary localizations of multiple myeloma.

Acknowledgements

We thank the nursing staff of the Department of Hematology, Hospital San Giuseppe Moscati, Taranto, Italy, who collaborated in the production of this work and especially:

Luciana Angela Talo for the patient management and Elisabetta Leggieri and Tamburrano Addolorata for the therapy management.

Conflict of interest

The authors declare no conflict of interest.

Author details

Giulia Palazzo[1*], Lara Aprile[1], Giacomo Cecere[1], Vito Pier Gagliardi[1], Alessandro Maggi[1], Antonella Prudenzano[2] and Patrizio Mazza[1]

1 Department of Hematology, Hospital San Giuseppe Moscati, Taranto, Italy

2 Laboratory of Hematology and Molecular Biology, Hospital San Giuseppe Moscati, Taranto, Italy

*Address all correspondence to: giuliapalazzo@libero.it

References

[1] Kilciksiz S, Karakoyun-Celik O, Agaoglu FY, Haydaroglu A. A review for solitary plasmacytoma of bone and extramedullary plasmacytoma. The Scientific World Journal [Internet]. Hindawi Limited; 2012;**2012**:1- 6. Available from: http://dx.doi.org/10.1100/2012/895765

[2] Zamagni E, Nanni C, Patriarca F, Englaro E, Castellucci P, Geatti O, et al. A prospective comparison of 18F-fluorodeoxyglucose positron emission tomography-computed tomography, magnetic resonance imaging and whole-body planar radiographs in the assessment of bone disease in newly diagnosed multiple myeloma. Haematologica [Internet]. Ferrata Storti Foundation (Haematologica); 2007 Jan 1;**92**(1):50-55. Available from: http://dx.doi.org/10.3324/haematol.10554

[3] Van Lammeren-Venema D, Regelink JC, Riphagen II, Zweegman S, Hoekstra OS, Zijlstra JM. 18F-fluoro-deoxyglucose positron emission tomography in assessment of myeloma-related bone disease: A systematic review. Cancer [Internet]. Wiley; 2011 Sep 1;**118**(8):1971-1981. Available from: http://dx.doi.org/10.1002/cncr.26467

[4] Dingli D, Ailawadhi S, Bergsagel PL, Buadi FK, Dispenzieri A, Fonseca R, et al. Therapy for Relapsed Multiple Myeloma. Mayo Clinic Proceedings [Internet]. Elsevier BV; 2017 Apr;**92**(4):578-598. Available from: http://dx.doi.org/10.1016/j.mayocp.2017.01.003

[5] Husnain M, Kurtin S, Barkett N, Riaz IB, Agarwal A. Refractory IgD multiple myeloma treated with daratumumab: A case report and literature review. Case Reports in Oncological Medicine [Internet]. Hindawi Limited; 2016;**2016**:1-4. Available from: http://dx.doi.org/10.1155/2016/2490168

Chapter 7

3D Models of Surrogate Multiple Myeloma Bone Marrow Microenvironments: Insights on Disease Pathophysiology and Patient-Specific Response to Drugs

Marina Ferrarini, Magda Marcatti, Fabio Ciceri and Elisabetta Ferrero

Abstract

Multiple Myeloma (MM) develops almost exclusively within the Bone Marrow (BM), highlighting the critical role of the microenvironment in conditioning disease progression and resistance to drugs. Indeed, while the therapeutic armamentarium for MM has significantly improved over the past 20 years, the disease remains ultimately incurable. This failure may depend on the high phenotypic and genetic heterogeneity of MM, but also on the paucity and inadequacy of two-dimensional (2D) conventional preclinical models in reproducing MM within the BM. In the present paper, we provide a brief updated overview on MM BM microenvironment. We then discuss newly developed preclinical models mimicking MM/microenvironment interactions, including three-dimensional (3D), gel-based, *in vitro* models and a novel *ex vivo* system of isolated tumor and stromal cells cultured in bioreactor. Potential applications of each model, relative to investigation of MM pathogenic mechanisms and prediction of the best drug/combination for each individual patient will be also evaluated.

Keywords: multiple myeloma, tumor microenvironment, 2D/3D culture models, 3D culture in bioreactor, drug testing, personalized therapy

1. Introduction

Multiple Myeloma (MM) is a B-cell tumor characterized by clonal proliferation of malignant plasma cells (PC) inside the bone marrow (BM), production of a monoclonal paraprotein and associated clinical features, including hypercalcemia, renal failure, anemia and lytic bone lesions (CRAB features) [1, 2].

MM is the second most common hematological malignancy and is responsible for approximately 20% of deaths from hematological tumors. Despite significant advances in therapy over the past two decades, the disease remains incurable, and more than 90% of MM patients eventually become refractory to therapy and relapse [1, 2].

MM develops along an evolutionary process, leading a normal PC to the premalignant state of monoclonal gammopathy of uncertain significance (MGUS), an intermediate asymptomatic but more advanced pre-malignant state referred to as smoldering MM (SMM) and finally to symptomatic MM [3–6]. This process is driven by the accumulation of cytogenetic modifications in PC. Indeed, while MM is still considered a single disease entity, it should be viewed as a collection of several different cytogenetically distinct PC tumors [7]. Cytogenetic abnormalities encompass translocations involving the immunoglobulin heavy chain (IgH) gene locus on chromosome 14q32 and hyperdiploidy (particularly trisomies), as initiating events [8]. IgH translocations include t(4;14), t(6;14), t(11;14), t(14;16) and t(14;20) translocations, which place the oncogenes Multiple Myeloma SET domain (MMSET)/ fibroblast growth factor receptor 3 (FGFR3), cyclin D3 (CCND3), CCND1, MAF, and MAFB, respectively, under the control of the strong enhancers of the Ig loci. This in turn leads to over-expression of cyclin D protein family members, ultimately driving G1/S checkpoint dysregulation [9, 10]. Hyperdiploidy, which is associated with the gain of the odd numbered chromosomes, including chromosome 3, 5, 7, 9, 11, 15, 19 and 21, also affects this checkpoint, implicating cyclin D dysregulation as an early and unifying oncogenic event in MM [9]. Subsequent studies demonstrated that other cytogenetic changes termed secondary cytogenetic abnormalities, including gain(1q), del(1p), del(17p), del(13), RAS mutations and secondary translocations involving MYC, arise along the disease course of MM, exacerbating the cell cycle dysregulation and driving further proliferation and disease progression [10, 11]. Patients carrying del(17p), t(4;14), t(14;16), t(14;20), gain(1q), or p53 mutation, particularly when in combination (double-hit and triple-hit myeloma), are considered affected by high-risk MM [11], and represent an area of unmet clinical need [8].

In addition to genetic abnormalities, a characteristic feature of myeloma cells is the requirement for an intimate relationship with the BM microenvironment, where plasma cells are nurtured in specialized niches that maintain their long-term survival. Indeed, BM components deeply influence many steps of tumor progression, such as MM proliferation and invasion, angiogenesis and drug resistance [12, 13].

The BM, where MM cells specifically home mainly through the CXCR4/CXCL12-SDF1α axis [14], provides a highly specialized microenvironment, which optimally "soils" neoplastic PC, and, in turn, is shaped by the interactions with the tumor [15, 16]. The BM microenvironment comprises two major compartments, *i.e.*, the cellular and the non-cellular compartment. The latter includes the extracellular matrix (ECM), consisting of collagen I to XI, fibronectin, glycoproteins, matrix proteoglycans and glycosaminoglycans, as well as the liquid milieu (cytokines, chemokines and growth factors). The cellular compartment consists of a series of components, including BM stromal cells (BMSC), hematopoietic cells, osteoclasts, osteoblasts, endothelial cells (EC), adipocytes and immune cells. Inside the BM milieu MM cells realize a complex interplay involving both cellular and ECM components through the engagement of adhesion molecules and the release of soluble factors, including cytokines, growth factors and exosomes [12]. Exosomes are extracellular membranous vesicles known to facilitate the transfer of biologically active molecules, including proteins and nucleic acids (particularly microRNAs -miRNAs), from the original producing cell to the target cell [17]. Exosomes are released by almost all cell types and, depending on their cargo, can induce target cell activation, proliferation/differentiation or death, thus playing a key role in the regulation of physiological as well as pathologic processes, including malignant transformation [17]. In MM, exosomes have been recently shown to reprogram the BM microenvironment, creating a niche for tumor PC and favoring their expansion and the onset of pharmacological resistance [18–20].

Another key feature of the BM microenvironment is hypoxia. In the BM, oxygen (O_2) tensions fluctuate throughout two specialized niches, the hypoxic endosteal niche and the oxygenated vascular niche, mapping areas with controlled, physiological O_2 gradients, instrumental to hematopoietic stem cells homeostasis [21]. BM homing is a common feature of hematological malignancies, that in proximity of hypoxic niches escape drug-inflicted apoptosis and acquire a drug-resistant phenotype. This is particularly true for MM that develops almost exclusively in the BM, where myeloma cells accumulation and the abnormal vasculature contribute to aggravate hypoxia. BM samples from MM patients as well as circulating MM cells are reported to have a hypoxic phenotype [22] and a strong stabilized expression of the hypoxia master regulator hypoxia-inducible factor (HIF)-1α protein [23]. Notably, HIF-1α suppression in myeloma cells blocks tumor growth *in vivo* and interferes negatively with angiogenesis and bone destruction [24]. In addition to conventional cell contact-dependent and -independent signaling pathways, hypoxia promotes MM survival and drug resistance through alternative mechanisms. Hypoxia is indeed a major regulator of exosomal content and angiogenesis in MM settings [25]. Moreover, hypoxia shifts the metabolic profile of MM cells toward elevated glycolysis and production of lactate, as a strategy to support energy requirement [26]. Notably, knockdown of lactate restores MM sensitivity to bortezomib, overall suggesting that targeting hypoxia and MM energy metabolism could alleviate drug resistance [26].

Overall, the cross-talk between MM cells and their BM microenvironment results in autocrine/paracrine loops of MM survival/proliferation and also promotes the "angiogenic switch", osteoclastogenesis, and defective immune functions [12, 13]. In particular, adhesion of MM cells to ECM components and to BMSC triggers classical survival signaling pathways including, but not limited to, the PI3K/AKT signaling pathway, anti-apoptotic signals and also the release of the pro-survival factor Interleukin (IL)-6 [27]. MM cells-BM interactions also play a key role in disease pathogenesis. In particular, new blood vessel formation is considered a hallmark of MM development and is supported by the histopathological evidence of increased microvessel density (MVD), surrogate parameter endowed with prognostic significance, in the BM of MM patients [28]. Angiogenesis, the sprouting of capillaries from existing blood vessels, is also suggested by the plethora of soluble angiogenic factors in the BM and in the peripheral blood (PB) samples from myeloma patients (vascular endothelial growth factor, VEGF; basic fibroblast growth factor, bFGF; angiopoietins, Angs) [29, 30], whose contribution to the process has been extensively reviewed [31]. Moreover, the finding of an elevated number of circulating endothelial precursor cells (EPC) in MM patients indicates that complementary modalities to build vessels, e.g., vasculogenesis, are engaged [31]. Finally, EC are by nature fine sensors of O_2 variations, and the hypoxic microenvironment inside the BM significantly contributes to the induction of the "angiogenic switch" and the maintenance of the pro-angiogenic profile through the transcription of HIF-1α [32].

MM plasma cells and BM stroma also contribute to the pathophysiology of MM-associated bone disease through the activation of signaling pathways regulating osteoclastogenesis, particularly the RANK/RANK-Ligand (RANK-L) and the Wnt pathway, and the release of osteoclast-activating factors, such as IL-1, IL-6, tumor necrosis factor (TNF)-α, IL-8 and Macrophage Inflammatory Protein (MIP)-1α. These factors, together with recently identified dysregulated miRNAs, determine osteoblast suppression with excessive osteoclastic resorption [33]. Finally, MM cells display a unique ability to evade immune surveillance through several mechanisms, including impairment of cytotoxic activity, induction of dendritic cell dysfunction and recruitment of regulatory cells [34].

2. 3D models of MM microenvironment for precision medicine

2.1 Therapeutic targeting of MM cells and their BM microenvironment: toward personalized therapy

Over the past 20 years, progressive understanding of the pathophysiology of MM has informed treatment paradigm and patients' outcome [35]. In particular, the introduction into the clinical practice of novel agents, such as proteasome inhibitors (PI) and immunomodulatory drugs (IMiDs), has prolonged median survival of MM patients from 3 to about 6 years, reaching approximatively 8 years in the subset of patients eligible to autologous stem cell transplantation (ASCT) [11].

The proteasome inhibitor bortezomib targets MM cells harnessing their dependency on the protein quality control pathway as a therapeutic target [36]. The ubiquitin-proteasome system represents a major mechanism for maintaining protein homeostasis, which is strictly required by normal antibody secreting PC, and particularly by MM PC [36]. Bortezomib causes an imbalance between proteasome degradative capacity and proteasome load, leading to the activation of the unfolded protein response, and ultimately to cell death *via* both intrinsic and extrinsic mechanisms of MM cell apoptosis [37]. Moreover, bortezomib affects viability of angiogenic EC [38], as well as bone turnover and osteoclast activity in the BM [39].

Given the key role of BM components in supporting MM cell proliferation, migration, survival and drug resistance, while also conferring immunosuppression, disrupting MM cells-BM interactions represents an alternative therapeutic strategy in MM. IMiDs, including thalidomide and its more potent derivatives lenalidomide and pomalidomide, have received Food and Drug Administration (FDA) approval for treatment of both newly diagnosed and relapsed/refractory MM [35]. IMiDs bind to cereblon (CRBN) and activate CRBN E3-ligase activity, causing the rapid ubiquitination and degradation of two specific B cell transcription factors, Ikaros (IKZF1) and Aiolos (IKZF3) [40, 41]. IMIDs thus exert direct cytotoxic effects on MM cells, including growth arrest, free radical-mediated DNA damage and caspase-8-mediated apoptosis; moreover, they modulate cytokine and growth factor secretion, inhibit angiogenesis, and, most importantly, upregulate T, NK, and NKT cytotoxicity, while downregulating regulatory T cells [42].

Over the disease course, however, MM cells acquire resistance to bortezomib and IMiDs through genetic and non-genetic mechanisms [36, 43]. To overcome resistance, second-generation PI (carfilzomib, ixazomib) and higher affinity CRBN E3-ligase modulators, such as iberdomide, have been developed [35, 36]. Alternative therapeutic approaches include: targeting epigenetic modifications *via* the Histone deacetylases (HDAC) inhibitors (panobinostat, ricolinostat); targeting the tumor-BM microenvironment interface *via* immune-based therapies, including monoclonal Antibodies (mAb) directed against MM surface antigens (elotuzumab and daratumumab, targeting SLAMF7 and CD38, respectively) and cellular therapies to boost MM- specific immunity, including adoptive T-cell therapy (ACT), engineered T-cell approaches and vaccines [35, 44]. Notably, progress in engineering technologies allowed for chimeric antigen receptor (CAR) T-cell approaches [45]. CAR are chimeric proteins that bring together the signaling moieties of the T cell receptor (TCR) complex and the variable domains of an Ab recognizing a tumor-associated antigen (in MM, most frequently the B cell maturation antigen –BCMA-, due to its selectivity for normal PC and MM cells) [35]. As a result, in the last decade, carfilzomib, pomalidomide, panobinostat, ixazomib, elotuzumab, daratumumab, isatuximab, and selinexor (a selective inhibitor of nuclear export of tumor suppressor proteins and growth factors) have received FDA approval for the treatment of relapsed MM, and are expected to improve outcomes further [11].

To date, therapy for an individual MM patient is selected based on clinical factors, such as age, performance status, comorbidities and eligibility for ASCT [46]. Given the high heterogeneity of the disease in terms of underlying molecular aberrations and clinical course, and also the growing armamentarium of currently available effective agents, this approach can be updated by the use of evidence-based algorithms [46], but it also needs to be implemented by incorporating prognostic and predictive biomarkers for survival and response to treatment [8]. Indeed, thanks to the progressive evolution and clinical utilization of molecular technologies, such as fluorescence in situ hybridization (FISH) and next-generation sequencing (NGS), we can foresee that in the near future the choice of therapy may include selection of targeted treatments based on the presence of specific molecular lesions, thus achieving personalized cancer care for MM patients [8]. Such treatments can be validated through randomized controlled clinical trials [8]; however, the development of reliable patient-specific pre-clinical models would also be valuable in the perspective of defining personalized, biologically based treatments for MM patients, while preventing ineffective therapy of resistant MM cells and unwanted toxicities [47].

2.2 *In vitro* models of cancer: moving from 2D to 3D

It is increasingly recognized that microenvironment plays a fundamental role in supporting tumor cell growth, survival and drug resistance; thus, experimental models of cancer should incorporate elements of the surrounding milieu to recreate and unveil the mechanisms that, at the molecular level, regulate the complex interplay between tumor cells and their embedding niche(s).

Traditional two-dimensional (2D) *in vitro* cultures, *i.e.*, static cultures of cells kept on flat, artificial surfaces, still represent the most popular models for *in vitro* studies. These culture systems have so far provided invaluable information on the basic molecular principles of cancer; it is becoming progressively clear, however, that they present severe limitations, since they fail to reproduce adequately morphology, behavior, and functions of normal and pathologic cell types and tissues [48]. It is now generally agreed that the generation of reliable and physiologically relevant *in vitro* tissue analogues, tumors included, should rely upon reproducing (or preserving) the specific characteristics of the native microenvironment. These encompass tissue-specific multiple cellularity and architecture, biochemical and mechanical cues, cell–cell and cell-ECM interactions and particularly the three-dimensionality (3D) [48, 49]. Indeed, since the pioneering work of Bissell and colleagues [50], several groups have extensively demonstrated that both normal and transformed cells maintained in traditional 2D culture significantly differ from cells kept in 3D culture in their biological behavior, gene expression profile and drug sensitivity [51–53].

Tissue engineering and regenerative medicine, originally aimed at developing biological substitutes of tissues or whole organs, have been subsequently extended to the generation of 3D platforms attempting to overcome the limitations of conventional culture models [54]. These platforms are based on different approaches, also depending on the aims to be addressed [49]. In particular, several experimental approaches rely on the use of polymeric substrates with tunable composition and stiffness, as scaffolds or hydrogel-based models. Scaffolds are key elements for the generation of 3D platforms, since they provide the mechanical support and physical composition for seeded cells to attach, grow and maintain their specialized functions. A suitable scaffold, such as a bone scaffold, must have favorable biocompatibility or cyto-compatibility and also adequate pore size and interconnectivity, in order to guarantee the growth, differentiation and proper penetration and distribution of different cell types [55]. Hydrogels are meant to mimic the ECM, and can be either natural or synthetic, the former commonly made with natural polymers (fibrinogen, hyaluronic acid, collagen, Matrigel and gelatin). Synthetic hydrogels are instead typically made with synthetic polymers (polyethylene glycol, polylactic acid, or poly-vinyl acetate) [49].

Scaffold-free models include spheroids and organoids. Spheroids are clusters of cells forced to assemble through hanging drop techniques or culture in bioreactor, taking advantage of the ability of cultured tumor cells to self-aggregate [56]. Spheroids derived from tumor cells, commonly referred to as tumorspheres, are typically monocultures, and therefore lack the multicellular identity that exists in a tumor *in vivo*. Organoids are cell aggregates, whose formation is driven by self-organizing, renewing stem cells, which differentiate *in vitro*, thus reproducing essential aspects of the parental organ [57]. Both structures are being exploited for drug testing, given their suitability for high throughput screening technologies. In particular, organoids grown from patients' tumor tissues (tumoroids) give rise to 3D structures with a multicellular identity that more faithfully recapitulate the complexity of the corresponding tumor they derive from, thus representing an advancement toward personalized medicine [58, 59]. The use of bioreactors and perfused microfluidic chambers adds to the complexity of the culture method, in that it allows a strict control of additional parameters, such as O_2, temperature, pH or nutrients [54]. Finally, the emerging 3D bioprinting technology has attracted increasing attention, based on its potential of manufacturing tissue-engineered compounds with well-defined 3D geometry [60]. In particular, these techniques are used to build tumor constructs via precise injection of living cells (both tumor and stroma) in functional biomaterials (bioinks), thus enabling the spatial–temporal control of molecular physical and chemical gradients [60, 61].

2.3 3D models of multiple myeloma

Since hematological malignancies with BM homing are supported by specialized niches, the complex BM architecture, together with cellular and molecular composition and interactions, needs to be replicated in engineered platforms to reproduce blood cancer behavior [54]. Indeed, while 2D cultures of established MM cell lines have been extensively used in high-throughput drug screening, they fail to reproduce BM microenvironment as well as the heterogeneity of MM patients' cells. The use of primary patient-derived MM cells in 2D monocultures or in co-cultures with stromal cells maintains the heterogeneity of the sample, but MM cell viability and functional interactions are often limited [47]. Finally, several animal models, which have been reviewed elsewhere [62–65], have been developed in order to support the growth of primary myeloma cells within a 3D microenvironment. While these models are more complex and therefore considered as more relevant, they are not representative of the human microenvironment. Within this context, 3D *in vitro/ex-vivo* human-derived culture systems are emerging as important tools to generate new approaches to the understanding of the molecular mechanisms of MM progression, essential prerequisites for the development of more effective interventional, diagnostic and prognostic strategies. The former often involve combination of multiple agents with the rationale that combining drugs with different mechanisms and targets could maximize their therapeutic efficacy [11]; this also should be taken into account in the design of 3D models for MM.

Herein we describe relevant 3D models of MM BM microenvironments that were generated exploiting different technical approaches, *i.e.*, gel and solid scaffolds –based 3D platforms, 3D models using microfluidics and 3D constructs cultured in bioreactor.

2.3.1 3D platforms using gel scaffolds

In 2008, Kirshner and co-workers reported the first *in vitro* reconstruction of the human MM BM microenvironment through a 3D model termed "rEnd-rBM". This was achieved by means of a proper overlay of matrix components, specifically collagen I/fibronectin to reconstruct endosteum-marrow junction (rEnd), and then a fibronectin/Matrigel mixture to create the recombinant BM (rBM) compartment, on which isolated cells from BM aspirates of MM patients were seeded [66]. Cells spontaneously redistributed throughout the gel-matrix 3D substrate, mimicking human BM architecture and BM-MM interactions, thus providing a powerful tool for understanding MM biology [66]. Strikingly, the reconstructed BM allowed the expansion of primary myeloma cells, including the putative cancer stem cell fraction embedded within the reconstructed endosteal niche. Moreover, the impact of anti-MM drugs, specifically bortezomib and melphalan, on distinct cellular compartments inside a 3D architecture could be assessed [66].

More recently, de la Puente et al. [67] developed a novel patient-derived 3D tissue-engineered BM culture model complexing BM supernatant of MM patients and autologous cells in a gel scaffold prepared from patient-derived plasma fibrinogen. The resulting construct contained all the growth factors, enzymes and cytokines naturally found in the MM microenvironment of an individual patient, better recapitulating the BM niche. The model reproduced the MM BM hypoxic gradients; moreover, it allowed *ex vivo* proliferation of primary MM cells for several weeks, and induced resistance in MM cells to various anti-myeloma drugs, such as carfilzomib and bortezomib [67].

An additional attempt to mimic the MM niche was performed by Jakubikova and colleagues [68], who developed a new 3D co-culture *ex-vivo* model of primary patient-derived MM cells and BMSC within a commercially available hydrogel (PuraMatrix). BMSC retained phenotypic and functional properties, together with lineage (osteoblastogenic) differentiation capacity. Notably, patient-derived MM cells showed increased proliferation and CXCR4 expression; moreover, BM-driven cell adhesion mediated drug resistance (CAM-DR) to both novel (IMiDs, bortezomib, carfilzomib) and conventional agents (doxorubicin, dexamethasone, melphalan) was observed in the 3D system and paralleled clinical resistance [68].

Finally, a further advancement was reported by Braham *et al* [69], who generated a novel *in vitro* 3D BM niche model by embedding mesenchymal stromal cells (MSC), EC and primary MM cells from patients inside a Matrigel matrix. The model harbored the characteristics of a representative tumor microenvironment, and was able to support long-term (up to 28 days) survival/proliferation of MM cells. The authors successfully exploited this tool to provide the first pre-clinical *in vitro* testing of immunotherapies on primary MM samples inside their tumor microenvironment. In fact, they showed that a novel class of engineered immune cells, *i.e.*, TCRα/β lymphocytes engineered to express tumor-specific Vγ9 VΔ2 TCRs (TEGs) [70], were able to infiltrate the 3D construct and efficiently kill MM cells [69].

2.3.2 3D platforms using silk scaffolds

Adopting a different strategy, based on the use of a strong, porous silk scaffold, MSC were induced to undergo osteogenic differentiation, recreating a mineralized 3D bone matrix [71]. The model allowed to reproduce proper MM-bone interactions in a standardized context and to study the MM-associated osteogenic process, demonstrating the negative impact of myeloma cells on normal bone homeostasis [71]. 3D silk scaffolds have also been employed by the same group to develop the first 3D, tissue-engineered BM adipose tissue (MAT) model, useful for elucidating the reciprocal interactions between MAT and tumor cells [72].

2.3.3 3D models using microfluidics

Recent technical advances include the tumor lab-on-a-chip, *in vitro* microfluidic devices that provide efficient platforms to recapitulate specific tumor traits, such as angiogenesis, hypoxia and tumor–stroma interactions, thus representing promising tools for personalized medicine [73]. In particular, functional hematopoietic niches have been constructed by culturing and perfusing bone in a sophisticated microfluidic -on-a-chip device [74]. These tools have been exploited to culture MM and BMSC lines, and to investigate MM chemoresistance to bortezomib, as well as the inducible activation of transcription factors [75]; their major limitations rely in the experimental procedure that does not incorporate the interplay between cancer cells the and surrounding stroma, critical to investigate MM progression [76].

2.3.4 3D culture of human MM tissue explants and of isolated MM cells in scaffolds in the microgravity-based RCCS™ bioreactor

The metabolic requirements of complex 3D cell constructs are substantially higher than those needed for the maintenance of traditional 2D cultures under static conditions. To meet this demand, dynamic bioreactors were primarily developed to optimize mass transfer, that is, gas/nutrient supply and waste elimination, all essential factors for preserving cell viability within large 3D cell/tissue masses. Among a wide array of fluid-dynamic bioreactors, the best conditions for long-term culture of functional 3D tissue-like bio-constructs and explants of various origin, including bone, were obtained with the introduction of the microgravity-based Rotary Cell Culture System (RCCS™, Synthecon Inc., USA) bioreactor [77–79] (a vast literature is available at http://www.synthecon.com). On this basis, we successfully employed the microgravity-based RCCS™ technology for the generation and long-term maintenance of viable human-derived MM tissue explants and 3D cell constructs. Our experimental procedure for culturing human tissue samples was firstly validated by using normal (skin and BM) and tumor biopsies [80]. Then, 3D culture of human MM tissue explants was found to maintain overall histo-architecture integrity and viability for up to two weeks. Moreover, the system was suitable for assessing the impact of drugs not only on MM cells, but also on angiogenic vessels, as evaluated through the assessment of MVD [80]. Finally, specialized functions of both MM cells and their microenvironment, including beta-2 microglobulin and cytokine release and metalloproteases activities, could be also assessed [80]. Overall, these observations suggest that 3D culture of MM tissues in bioreactor is feasible and can be potentially exploited as a novel translational tool for patient-specific drug testing.

A major limitation to a systematic pre-clinical use of this approach, however, is represented by the restricted availability of human MM biopsies for tissue culture, besides those obtained for diagnostic purposes. To overcome this limitation, we have recently established a novel procedure based on the reconstruction of a 3D surrogate MM BM microenvironment [81]. This model relies on the co-seeding of MM cells and stroma inside a gelatin sponge, which is subsequently cultured in bioreactor. **Figure 1** schematically represents the procedure developed to generate MM BM surrogate microenvironments, as well as the information that can be obtained through the analysis of both repopulated scaffolds and culture supernatants. Myeloma cell lines engaged contacts with stromal cells, EC and osteoblasts, as assessed by histochemical and electron-microscopic analyses. Consistently,

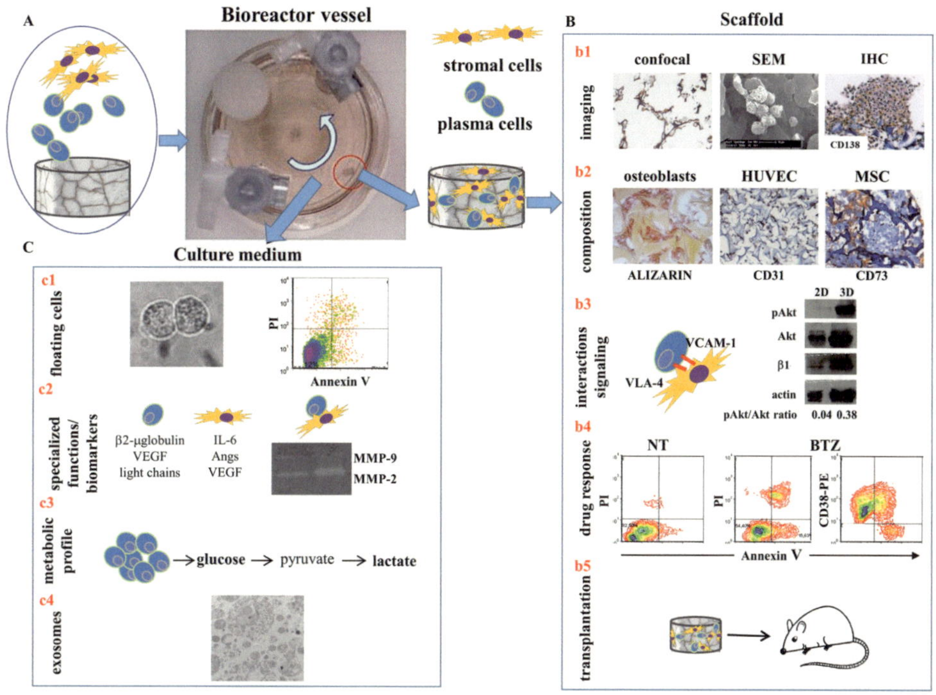

Figure 1.
Information obtainable from 3D MM- BM stroma co-culture in bioreactor. (A) Schematic representation of the experimental procedure: Selected elements of the BM milieu (as in b2, along with lineage-specific markers) and plasma cells are sequentially seeded into the scaffold and kept in culture in bioreactor. (B) Scaffolds retrieved from the bioreactor at the end of the culture period can be: b1: Either fixed or frozen and submitted to imaging by confocal, scanning electromicroscopy (SEM) or immunohistochemistry (IHC) analyses; b3: Lysed and processed for Western blot analysis (right) for the expression of integrins and signaling pathways resulting from tumor-stroma interactions, schematically represented in (left); b4: Enzymatically dissociated to single cells for quantification, characterization and assessment of drug-induced apoptosis by FACS analysis; b5: Ectopically transplanted into mice. (C) Culture medium withdrawn from the bioreactor can be processed to: c1: Characterize floating MM cells, reminiscent of circulating MM cells; c2: Assess specialized functions, attributable to both stroma and MM cells; c3: Determine the content of glycolitic metabolites; c4: Quantify and characterize the content of exosomes. Abbreviations: VEGF = vascular endothelial growth factor; IL = interleukin; Ang = angiopoietin; MMP = matrix metalloproteases; HUVEC = human umbilical vein endothelial cells; MSC = mesenchymal stromal cells; pAkt = phospho-AKT; β1 = β1 integrin; PI = propidium iodide; PE = phycoerythrin; BTZ = bortezomib.

pro-survival signaling and also CAM-DR, particularly through the engagement of the integrin VLA-4 by its counter-receptor VCAM1 [82], were significantly higher in 3D than in 2D parallel co-cultures. Soluble factor-mediated drug resistance could be also appreciated in 3D co-cultures. The system was then successfully applied to co-cultures of primary myeloma cells-primary myeloma BMSC and EC, allowing the functionalization of myeloma-stroma interactions and MM cell long-term survival. Finally, the impact of bortezomib on myeloma cells and on specialized functions of the microenvironment could be evaluated. Significantly, the model also showed the potential for assessing clonal evolution *ex-vivo*. In fact, MM cells obtained from a high-risk patient actively proliferated in bioreactor, paralleling the elevated proliferation index observed in the patient's bone biopsy, and anticipated the expansion of a clone that ultimately dominated *in vivo,* thus predicting the clinical outcome [81].

Further studies validated the use of the model for additional purposes, including investigation on novel pathogenic interactions and preclinical drug testing. In particular, modeling the interaction between the receptor tyrosine kinase ROR2 and its ligand WNT5A in bioreactor allowed identifying this pathway as crucial in the adhesion of MM cells to the BM microenvironment, and as a potential therapeutic target for the large subgroup of MM patients whose cancer cells show ROR2 overexpression [83]. Moreover, the use of surrogate MM microenvironments in bioreactor complemented studies performed both *in vitro* and in animal models to exploit the DNA damage response as a novel therapeutic strategy for MM. In particular, the combination of drugs causing ATR inhibition (the compound VX-970) and melphalan, a widely used alkylating agent eliciting inter-strand cross-links, proved dramatically effective, thus paving the way to future clinical testing [84]. An additional advantage provided by culture in bioreactor of MM samples or surrogate MM BM on scaffolds is that the well-preserved material can be frozen to create a biobank suitable to serially test patient-specific sensitivity, as for organoids [59].

Our surrogate BM microenvironment could also be exploited for other hematological malignancies infiltrating the BM niches. In particular, Chronic Lymphocytic Leukemia (CLL) is characterized by a progressive expansion of clonal CD5+ B lymphocytes that dynamically traffic from PB to the more protective BM and secondary lymphoid organs, where they acquire an aggressive phenotype and drug resistance [13]. In this context, new targeted therapies, namely kinase inhibitors (KI), have been developed to promote mobilization of leukemic cells from the hosting tissues into the PB, where they may re-acquire sensitivity to drug-induced apoptosis [85]. Our 3D surrogate BM microenvironment was exploited to recreate the niche-specific interplay involved in CLL cells homing/mobilization, showing that distinct molecular interactions, in particular through the HS1 cytoskeletal protein, were reproduced [86]. We could demonstrate that HS1 conversion from the active to the inactive form, promoted by the KI ibrutinib, was able to regulate CLL cells retention inside- and mobilization from- scaffolds. This indicates that the model may serve as a good platform to unveil the mechanisms underlying tumor cells dissemination and to predict the impact of mobilizing agents [86], conceivably also in MM.

The same *in vitro* 3D dynamic culture system in RCCS™ bioreactor was used by Bonomi et al. [87] to generate spheroids of myeloma cells co-cultured with BMSCs. By that mean, the authors demonstrated that BMSCs loaded with Paclitaxel (PTX) could serve as a 'Trojan horse' to vehicle and deliver *in situ* anti-tumor agents in amounts sufficient to affect tumor growth. The inhibitory activity of PTX-primed BMSCs was comparable to that of PTX alone, showing that the loaded-BMSC strategy could be exploited to deliver drugs into the BM.

3. Conclusions and perspectives

The BM, where MM cells home, survive and accumulate, represents a complex and highly specialized tumor microenvironment, making the development of engineered 3D platforms of MM a challenging task. Indeed, in addition to a series of distinct ECM and cellular components, the BM microenvironment comprises several factors, including specialized niches, hypoxic gradients, vascularization and a mineralized matrix, all to be taken into account to faithfully recapitulate the native tumor. Nevertheless, already available pre-clinical models of MM represent a remarkable example of translational cancer research [88], potentially covering issues ranging from high- throughput drug assessment/screening to investigation on MM pathophysiology and patient-tailored drug testing aimed at precision oncology. **Table 1** summarizes the main features of the previously described 3D models of MM BM microenvironments, together with their suitability, in our view, to different purposes. In particular, microfluidic systems could be exploited for drug screening/development with high-throughput potential, in that they can be miniaturized to cope with the limited biological starting material

3D model	Reference	Composition	Drug tested	Drug screening	Precision Oncology	MM biology
Gel scaffold	Kirshner et al., 2008 [66]	ECM components + MM BM aspirates	Melphalan, Btz	—	+	+
Gel scaffold	de la Puente et al., 2015 [67]	Fibrin gel + MM cells + BMSC/EC	Btz, Cfz	—	+	+
Gel scaffold	Jakubikova et al., 2016 [68]	PuraMatrix hydrogel +primary MM cells + BMSC	iMiDs, Btz, Cfz DOXO, DEX, Melphalan	—	+	+
Gel scaffold	Braham et al., 2018 [69]	Matrigel+ BMSC +EC + MM cells	TEGs (αβ T cells expressing Vγ9 Vδ2 TCRs)	—	+	+
Solid scaffold	Reagan et al., 2014 [71]	Silk scaffold+ MM cells +BMSC/EC	Btz	—	+	+
Solid scaffold	Fairfield et al., 2019 [72]	Silk scaffold+ MM cell lines+ BMSC	none	—	—	+
Microfluidics	Young et al., 2012 [75]	Microchambers +MM cell lines +BMSC	Btz	+	+	—
Bioreactor-based	Belloni et al., 2018 [81]	Gelatin scaffolds populated by MM cell lines/primary MM cells + BMSC/EC/OB cultured in bioreactor	Btz, Melphalan, DEX	—	+	+
Bioreactor-based	Bonomi et al., 2017 [87]	Spheroids of MM cell lines + BMSC cultured in bioreactor	Paclitaxel	—	+	—

Abbreviations: ECM = extracellular matrix; MM = Multiple Myeloma; BM = Bone Marrow; BMSC = BM stromal cells; EC = endothelial cells; OB = osteoblasts; Btz = bortezomib; Cfz = carfilzomib; iMIDs = immunomodulatory drugs; DOXO = doxorubicin; DEX = dexamethasone.

Table 1.
Summary of different experimental approaches to model the MM BM microenvironment: Potential applications.

than can be obtained from MM patients' samples. Most of the 3D platforms can be used in principle to test a selected range of drugs in a more precise microenvironmental context, in the perspective of personalized therapy and prediction of resistance. Finally, complex 3D technologies, such as bioreactor-based dynamic culture systems, while less easy to handle, can be tuned to recreate proper MM milieu and interactions, thus being suitable to investigation on MM pathophysiology and the mechanisms of drugs. Future efforts combining interdisciplinary basic and technical proficiencies, in particular related to tissue engineering, new biomaterials and advanced imaging techniques [48, 89], are expected to generate fully-humanized, simple, cost-effective, reliable and standardized models that can be more widely employed in the pre-clinical setting, particularly in high-risk and in relapsed/resistant MM patients.

In addition to the purpose of precision oncology, 3D platforms can be applied to explore novel pathogenic cues. In particular, several matters that are object of intense investigation, including hypoxia and tumor metabolism, as well as the contribution of exosomes and miRNAs in the interactions between tumor and its co-evolving microenvironment, could be fruitfully and more precisely investigated applying advanced technological approaches, as already done in different settings (**Figure 1** and [90, 91]). Further exploitation of the SCID/scaffold model, based on the transplantation of 3D bone-like polymeric scaffolds into immunocompromised mice, can also be envisaged to dissect biological events in primary MM cells engrafted inside a human BM microenvironment, as well as their response to drug in a *in vivo* context (**Figure 1B**). Additional future directions include the development and implementation of new technologies, such as microfluidic and bioprinting techniques, to further add to the complexity of *in vitro* surrogate MM BM microenvironments, particularly with regard to MM associated angiogenesis and components of the immune system.

Acknowledgements

We wish to thank Dr. Antonello Villa (Università Milano Bicocca, Milan, Italy) for his outstanding contribution in generating confocal, immunohistochemistry and electron-microscopy images; Dr. Daniela Belloni (Division of Experimental Oncology, San Raffaele Scientific Institute, Milan, Italy) for developing the 3D model in bioreactor and performing experiments; Prof Federico Caligaris-Cappio (Italian Association for Cancer Research-AIRC) and Dr. Giovanni Tonon (Division of Experimental Oncology, San Raffaele Scientific Institute, Milan, Italy) for helpful discussion and unceasing support; Prof. Paolo Ghia (Division of Experimental Oncology, San Raffaele Scientific Institute, Milan, Italy) for precious insights.

Funding information

Papers from our group cited in this chapter were partially supported by the AIRC 5x1000 Project n 9965 (to Prof Federico Caligaris Cappio) and its extension (to Prof Paolo Ghia).

Conflict of interest

The authors declare no Conflict of Interest.

Author details

Marina Ferrarini[1*], Magda Marcatti[2], Fabio Ciceri[2] and Elisabetta Ferrero[1*]

1 B-Cell Neoplasia Unit, Division of Experimental Oncology, San Raffaele Scientific Institute, Milan, Italy

2 Department of Hematology and Stem Cell Transplantation, San Raffaele Scientific Institute, Milan, Italy

*Address all correspondence to: ferrarini.marina@hsr.it
and ferrero.elisabetta@hsr.it

References

[1] Rajkumar SV, Dimopoulos MA, Palumbo A, Blade J, Merlini G, Mateos MV, Kumar S, Hillengass J, Kastritis E, Richardson P, Landgren O, Paiva B, Dispenzieri A, Weiss B, LeLeu X, Zweegman S, Lonial S, Rosinol L, Zamagni E, Jagannath S, Sezer O, Kristinsson SY, Caers J, Usmani SZ, Lahuerta JJ, Johnsen HE, Beksac M, Cavo M, Goldschmidt H, Terpos E, Kyle RA, Anderson KC, Durie BG, Miguel JF. International Myeloma Working Group updated criteria for the diagnosis of multiple myeloma. Lancet Oncol. 2014;15(12):e538-48. DOI: 10.1016/S1470-2045(14)70442-5.

[2] Kumar SK, Rajkumar V, Kyle RA, van Duin M, Sonneveld P, Mateos MV, Gay F, Anderson KC. Multiple myeloma. Nat Rev Dis Primers. 2017;3:17046. DOI: 10.1038/nrdp.2017.46.

[3] Chesi M, Bergsagel PL, Brents LA, Smith CM, Gerhard DS, Kuehl WM. Dysregulation of cyclin D1 by translocation into an IgH gamma switch region in two multiple myeloma cell lines. Blood. 1996;88(2):674-81

[4] Fonseca R, Debes-Marun CS, Picken EB, Dewald GW, Bryant SC, Winkler JM, Blood E, Oken MM, Santana-Dávila R, González-Paz N, Kyle RA, Gertz MA, Dispenzieri A, Lacy MQ, Greipp PR. The recurrent IgH translocations are highly associated with nonhyperdiploid variant multiple myeloma. Blood. 2003;102(7):2562-7. DOI: 10.1182/blood-2003-02-0493.

[5] González D, van der Burg M, García-Sanz R, Fenton JA, Langerak AW, González M, van Dongen JJ, San Miguel JF, Morgan GJ. Immunoglobulin gene rearrangements and the pathogenesis of multiple myeloma. Blood. 2007;110(9):3112-21. DOI: 10.1182/blood-2007-02-069625.

[6] Pawlyn C, Morgan GJ. Evolutionary biology of high-risk multiple myeloma. Nat Rev Cancer. 2017;17(9):543-556. DOI: 10.1038/nrc.2017.63.

[7] Kumar SK, Rajkumar SV. The multiple myelomas - current concepts in cytogenetic classification and therapy. Nat Rev Clin Oncol. 2018;15(7):409-421. DOI: 10.1038/s41571-018-0018-y.

[8] Pawlyn C, Davies FE. Toward personalized treatment in multiple myeloma based on molecular characteristics. Blood. 2019;133(7):660-675. DOI: 10.1182/blood-2018-09-825331.

[9] Bergsagel PL, Kuehl WM, Zhan F, Sawyer J, Barlogie B, Shaughnessy J Jr. Cyclin D dysregulation: an early and unifying pathogenic event in multiple myeloma. Blood. 2005;106(1):296-303. DOI: 10.1182/blood-2005-01-0034.

[10] Morgan GJ, Walker BA, Davies FE. The genetic architecture of multiple myeloma. Nat Rev Cancer. 2012;12(5):335-48. DOI: 10.1038/nrc3257.

[11] Rajkumar SV. Multiple myeloma: 2020 update on diagnosis, risk-stratification and management. Am J Hematol. 2020 May;95(5):548-567. DOI: 10.1002/ajh.25791.

[12] Hideshima T, Mitsiades C, Tonon G, Richardson PG, Anderson KC. Understanding multiple myeloma pathogenesis in the bone marrow to identify new therapeutic targets. Nat Rev Cancer. 2007:585-98. DOI: 10.1038/nrc2189.

[13] Burger JA, Ghia P, Rosenwald A, Caligaris-Cappio F. The microenvironment in mature B-cell malignancies: a target for new treatment strategies. Blood. 2009;114(16):3367-75. DOI: 10.1182/blood-2009-06-225326.

[14] Alsayed Y, Ngo H, Runnels J, Leleu X, Singha UK, Pitsillides CM,

Spencer JA, Kimlinger T, Ghobrial JM, Jia X, Lu G, Timm M, Kumar A, Côté D, Veilleux I, Hedin KE, Roodman GD, Witzig TE, Kung AL, Hideshima T, Anderson KC, Lin CP, Ghobrial IM. Mechanisms of regulation of CXCR4/SDF-1 (CXCL12)-dependent migration and homing in multiple myeloma. Blood. 2007;109(7):2708-17. DOI: 10.1182/blood-2006-07-035857.

[15] Tripodo C, Sangaletti S, Piccaluga PP, Prakash S, Franco G, Borrello I, Orazi A, Colombo MP, Pileri SA. The bone marrow stroma in hematological neoplasms--a guilty bystander. Nat Rev Clin Oncol. 2011;8(8):456-66. DOI: 10.1038/nrclinonc.2011.31.

[16] Vacca A, Ribatti D. Bone marrow angiogenesis in multiple myeloma. Leukemia. 2006;20(2):193-9. DOU: 10.1038/sj.leu.2404067.

[17] Boyiadzis M, Whiteside TL. The emerging roles of tumor-derived exosomes in hematological malignancies. Leukemia. 2017;31(6):1259-1268. DOI: 10.1038/leu.2017.91.

[18] Roccaro AM, Sacco A, Maiso P, Azab AK, Tai YT, Reagan M, Azab F, Flores LM, Campigotto F, Weller E, Anderson KC, Scadden DT, Ghobrial IM. BM mesenchymal stromal cell-derived exosomes facilitate multiple myeloma progression. J Clin Invest. 2013;123(4):1542-55. DOI: 10.1172/JCI66517

[19] Colombo M, Giannandrea D, Lesma E, Basile A, Chiaramonte R. Extracellular Vesicles Enhance Multiple Myeloma Metastatic Dissemination. Int J Mol Sci. 2019;20(13):3236. DOI: 10.3390/ijms20133236.

[20] Raimondo S, Urzì O, Conigliaro A, Raimondi L, Amodio N, Alessandro R. Emerging Insights on the Biological Impact of Extracellular Vesicle-Associated ncRNAs in Multiple Myeloma. Noncoding RNA. 2020;6(3):30. DOI: 10.3390/ncrna6030030.

[21] Muz B, de la Puente P, Azab F, Luderer M, Azab AK. The role of hypoxia and exploitation of the hypoxic environment in hematologic malignancies. Mol Cancer Res. 2014;12(10):1347-54. DOI: 10.1158/1541-7786.MCR-14-0028.

[22] Colla S, Storti P, Donofrio G, Todoerti K, Bolzoni M, Lazzaretti M, Abeltino M, Ippolito L, Neri A, Ribatti D, Rizzoli V, Martella E, Giuliani N. Low bone marrow oxygen tension and hypoxia-inducible factor-1α overexpression characterize patients with multiple myeloma: role on the transcriptional and proangiogenic profiles of CD138(+) cells. Leukemia. 2010;24(11):1967-70. DOI: 10.1038/leu.2010.193.

[23] Semenza GL. Hypoxia-inducible factors in physiology and medicine. Cell. 2012;148(3):399-408. DOI: 10.1016/j.cell.2012.01.021.

[24] Storti P, Bolzoni M, Donofrio G, Airoldi I, Guasco D, Toscani D, Martella E, Lazzaretti M, Mancini C, Agnelli L, Patrene K, Maiga S, Franceschi V, Colla S, Anderson J, Neri A, Amiot M, Aversa F, Roodman GD, Giuliani N. Hypoxia-inducible factor (HIF)-1alpha suppression in myeloma cells blocks tumoral growth in vivo inhibiting angiogenesis and bone destruction. Leukemia. 2013 27(8):1697-1706. DOI: 10.1038/leu.2012.190.

[25] Ohyashiki JH, Umezu T, Ohyashiki K. Exosomes promote bone marrow angiogenesis in hematologic neoplasia: the role of hypoxia. Curr Opin Hematol. 2016;23(3):268-73. DOI: 10.1097/MOH.0000000000000235.

[26] Maiso P, Huynh D, Moschetta M, Sacco A, Aljawai Y, Mishima Y, Asara JM, Roccaro AM, Kimmelman AC, Ghobrial IM. Metabolic signature

identifies novel targets for drug resistance in multiple myeloma. Cancer Res. 2015 May 15;75(10): 2071-82. DOI: 10.1158/0008-5472. CAN-14-3400.

[27] Gunn WG, Conley A, Deininger L, Olson SD, Prockop DJ, Gregory CA. A crosstalk between myeloma cells and marrow stromal cells stimulates production of DKK1 and interleukin-6: a potential role in the development of lytic bone disease and tumor progression in multiple myeloma. Stem Cells. 2006;24(4):986-91. DOI: 10.1634/ stemcells.2005-0220.

[28] Sezer O, Niemöller K, Eucker J, Jakob C, Kaufmann O, Zavrski I, Dietel M, Possinger K. Bone marrow microvessel density is a prognostic factor for survival in patients with multiple myeloma. Ann Hematol. 2000;79(10):574-7. DOI: 10.1007/ s002770000236.

[29] Ribatti D, Nico B, Vacca A. Multiple myeloma as a model for the role of bone marrow niches in the control of angiogenesis. Int Rev Cell Mol Biol. 2015;314:259-82. DOI: 10.1016/ bs.ircmb.2014.10.004.

[30] Belloni D, Marcatti M, Ponzoni M, Ciceri F, Veschini L, Corti A, Caligaris Cappio F, Ferrarini M, Ferrero E. Angiopoietin-2 in Bone Marrow milieu promotes Multiple Myeloma-associated angiogenesis. Exp Cell Res. 2015;330(1):1-12. DOI: 10.1016/j. yexcr.2014.10.017.

[31] Vacca A, Ribatti D. Bone marrow angiogenesis in multiple myeloma. Leukemia. 2006;20(2):193-9. DOI: 10.1038/sj.leu.2404067.

[32] Ferrarini M, Ferrero E. Proteasome inhibitors and modulators of angiogenesis in multiple myeloma. Curr Med Chem. 2011;18(34):5185-95. DOI: 10.2174/092986711798184316.

[33] Raimondi L, De Luca A, Giavaresi G, Raimondo S, Gallo A, Taiana E, Alessandro R, Rossi M, Neri A, Viglietto G, Amodio N. Non-Coding RNAs in Multiple Myeloma Bone Disease Pathophysiology. Noncoding RNA. 2020;6(3):E37. DOI: 10.3390/ncrna6030037.

[34] Kawano Y, Moschetta M, Manier S, Glavey S, Görgün GT, Roccaro AM, Anderson KC, Ghobrial IM. Targeting the bone marrow microenvironment in multiple myeloma. Immunol Rev. 2015;263(1):160-72. DOI: 10.1111/ imr.12233.

[35] Gulla A, Anderson KC. Multiple myeloma: the (r)evolution of current therapy and a glance into future. Haematologica. 2020 Jul 23:haematol.2020.247015. DOI: 10.3324/ haematol.2020.247015.

[36] Gandolfi S, Laubach JP, Hideshima T, Chauhan D, Anderson KC, Richardson PG. The proteasome and proteasome inhibitors in multiple myeloma. Cancer Metastasis Rev. 2017;36(4):561-584. DOI: 10.1007/ s10555-017-9707-8.

[37] Bianchi G, Oliva L, Cascio P, Pengo N, Fontana F, Cerruti F, Orsi A, Pasqualetto E, Mezghrani A, Calbi V, Palladini G, Giuliani N, Anderson KC, Sitia R, Cenci S. The proteasome load versus capacity balance determines apoptotic sensitivity of multiple myeloma cells to proteasome inhibition. Blood. 2009;113(13):3040-9. DOI: 10.1182/blood-2008-08-172734.

[38] Belloni D, Veschini L, Foglieni C, Dell'Antonio G, Caligaris-Cappio F, Ferrarini M, Ferrero E. Bortezomib induces autophagic death in proliferating human endothelial cells. Exp Cell Res. 2010;316(6):1010-8. DOI: 10.1016/j.yexcr.2009.

[39] Hideshima T, Anderson KC. Biologic impact of proteasome inhibition in

multiple myeloma cells-from the aspects of preclinical studies. Semin Hematol. 2012;49(3):223-7. DOI: 10.1053/j.seminhematol.2012.04.006.

[40] Krönke J, Udeshi ND, Narla A, Grauman P, Hurst SN, McConkey M, Svinkina T, Heckl D, Comer E, Li X, Ciarlo C, Hartman E, Munshi N, Schenone M, Schreiber SL, Carr SA, Ebert BL. Lenalidomide causes selective degradation of IKZF1 and IKZF3 in multiple myeloma cells. Science. 2014;343(6168):301-5. DOI: 10.1126/science.1244851.

[41] Lu G, Middleton RE, Sun H, Naniong M, Ott CJ, Mitsiades CS, Wong KK, Bradner JE, Kaelin WG Jr. The myeloma drug lenalidomide promotes the cereblon-dependent destruction of Ikaros proteins. Science. 2014;343(6168):305-9. DOI: 10.1126/science.1244917.

[42] Davies F, Baz R. Lenalidomide mode of action: linking bench and clinical findings. Blood Rev. 2010;24 Suppl 1:S13-9. DOI: 10.1016/S0268-960X(10)70004-7.

[43] Martinez-Høyer S, Karsan A. Mechanisms of lenalidomide sensitivity and resistance. Exp Hematol. 2020:S0301-472X(20)30561-0. DOI: 10.1016/j.exphem.2020.09.196. Epub ahead of print.

[44] Boussi L, Niesvizky R. Advances in immunotherapy in multiple myeloma. Curr Opin Oncol. 2017;29(6):460-466. DOI: 10.1097/CCO.0000000000000407.

[45] Norelli M, Casucci M, Bonini C, Bondanza A. Clinical pharmacology of CAR-T cells: Linking cellular pharmacodynamics to pharmacokinetics and antitumor effects. Biochim Biophys Acta. 2016;1865(1):90-100. DOI: 10.1016/j.bbcan.2015.12.001.

[46] Rajkumar SV, Kumar S. Multiple myeloma current treatment algorithms. Blood Cancer J. 2020;10(9):94. DOI: 10.1038/s41408-020-00359-2.

[47] Papadimitriou K, Kostopoulos IV, Tsopanidou A, Orologas-Stavrou N, Kastritis E, Tsitsilonis O, Dimopoulos MA, Terpos E. Ex Vivo Models Simulating the Bone Marrow Environment and Predicting Response to Therapy in Multiple Myeloma. Cancers (Basel). 2020;12(8):2006. DOI: 10.3390/cancers12082006.

[48] Pampaloni F, Reynaud EG, Stelzer EH. The third dimension bridges the gap between cell culture and live tissue. Nat Rev Mol Cell Biol. 2007;8(10):839-45. DOI: 10.1038/nrm2236.

[49] Jensen C, Teng Y. Is It Time to Start Transitioning From 2D to 3D Cell Culture? Front Mol Biosci. 2020;7:33. DOI: 10.3389/fmolb.2020.00033.

[50] Lee GY, Kenny PA, Lee EH, Bissell MJ. Three-dimensional culture models of normal and malignant breast epithelial cells. Nat Methods. 2007;4(4):359-65. DOI: 10.1038/nmeth1015.

[51] Chang TT, Hughes-Fulford M. Monolayer and spheroid culture of human liver hepatocellular carcinoma cell line cells demonstrate distinct global gene expression patterns and functional phenotypes. Tissue Eng Part A. 2009;15(3):559-67. DOI: 10.1089/ten.tea.2007.0434.

[52] Pickl M, Ries CH. Comparison of 3D and 2D tumor models reveals enhanced HER2 activation in 3D associated with an increased response to trastuzumab. Oncogene. 2009;28(3):461-8. DOI: 10.1038/onc.2008.394.

[53] Riedl A, Schlederer M, Pudelko K, Stadler M, Walter S, Unterleuthner D, Unger C, Kramer N, Hengstschläger M, Kenner L, Pfeiffer D, Krupitza G, Dolznig H. Comparison of cancer cells

in 2D vs 3D culture reveals differences in AKT-mTOR-S6K signaling and drug responses. J Cell Sci. 2017;130(1):203-218. DOI: 10.1242/jcs.188102.

[54] Clara-Trujillo S, Gallego Ferrer G, Gómez Ribelles JL. In Vitro Modeling of Non-Solid Tumors: How Far Can Tissue Engineering Go? Int J Mol Sci. 2020;21(16):5747. DOI: 10.3390/ijms21165747.

[55] Carletti E, Motta A, Migliaresi C. Scaffolds for tissue engineering and 3D cell culture. Methods Mol Biol. 2011;695:17-39. doi: 10.1007/978-1-60761-984-0_2

[56] Hirschhaeuser F, Menne H, Dittfeld C, West J, Mueller-Klieser W, Kunz-Schughart LA. Multicellular tumor spheroids: an underestimated tool is catching up again. J Biotechnol. 2010;148(1):3-15. DOI: 10.1016/j.jbiotec.2010.01.012.

[57] Yin X, Mead BE, Safaee H, Langer R, Karp JM, Levy O. Engineering Stem Cell Organoids. Cell Stem Cell. 2016;18(1):25-38. DOI: 10.1016/j.stem.2015.12.005.

[58] Smith AR, Kuo CJ. Organoids lead the cancer attack. Nat Med. 2017;23(12):1399-1400. DOI: 10.1038/nm.4454.

[59] Drost J, Clevers H. Organoids in cancer research. Nat Rev Cancer. 2018;18(7):407-418. DOI: 10.1038/s41568-018-0007-6.

[60] Datta P, Dey M, Ataie Z, Unutmaz D, Ozbolat IT. 3D bioprinting for reconstituting the cancer microenvironment. NPJ Precis Oncol. 2020;4:18. DOI: 10.1038/s41698-020-0121-2.

[61] Meng F, Meyer CM, Joung D, Vallera DA, McAlpine MC, Panoskaltsis-Mortari A. 3D Bioprinted In Vitro Metastatic Models via Reconstruction of Tumor Microenvironments. Adv Mater. 2019;31(10):e1806899. DOI: 10.1002/adma.201806899.

[62] Vanderkerken K, Asosingh K, Croucher P, Van Camp B. Multiple myeloma biology: lessons from the 5TMM models. Immunol Rev. 2003;194:196-206. DOI: 10.1034/j.1600-065x.2003.00035.x.

[63] Ferrarini M, Mazzoleni G, Steimberg N, Belloni D, Ferrero E. Innovative models to assess Multiple Myeloma biology and the impact of drugs. In Hajek R, editor. Multiple Myeloma – A quick reflection on the fast progress. InTechOpen; 2013, p 39-60. DOI:10.5772/54312.

[64] Rossi M, Botta C, Arbitrio M, Grembiale RD, Tagliaferri P, Tassone P. Mouse models of multiple myeloma: technologic platforms and perspectives. Oncotarget. 2018;9(28):20119-20133. DOI: 10.18632/oncotarget.24614.

[65] Cooke RE, Koldej R, Ritchie D. Immunotherapeutics in Multiple Myeloma: How Can Translational Mouse Models Help? J Oncol. 2019;2019:2186494. DOI:10.1155/2019/2186494.

[66] Kirshner J, Thulien KJ, Martin LD, Debes Marun C, Reiman T, Belch AR, Pilarski LM. A unique three-dimensional model for evaluating the impact of therapy on multiple myeloma. Blood. 2008;112(7):2935-45. DOI: 10.1182/blood-2008-02-142430.

[67] de la Puente P, Muz B, Gilson RC, Azab F, Luderer M, King J, Achilefu S, Vij R, Azab AK. 3D tissue-engineered bone marrow as a novel model to study pathophysiology and drug resistance in multiple myeloma. Biomaterials. 2015;73:70-84. DOI: 10.1016/j.biomaterials.2015.09.017.

[68] Jakubikova J, Cholujova D, Hideshima T, Gronesova P,

Soltysova A, Harada T, Joo J, Kong SY, Szalat RE, Richardson PG, Munshi NC, Dorfman DM, Anderson KC. A novel 3D mesenchymal stem cell model of the multiple myeloma bone marrow niche: biologic and clinical applications. Oncotarget. 2016;7(47):77326-77341. DOI: 10.18632/oncotarget.12643.

[69] Braham MVJ, Minnema MC, Aarts T, Sebestyen Z, Straetemans T, Vyborova A, Kuball J, Öner FC, Robin C, Alblas J. Cellular immunotherapy on primary multiple myeloma expanded in a 3D bone marrow niche model. Oncoimmunology. 2018;7(6):e1434465. DOI: 10.1080/2162402X.2018.1434465.

[70] Marcu-Malina V, Heijhuurs S, van Buuren M, Hartkamp L, Strand S, Sebestyen Z, Scholten K, Martens A, Kuball J. Redirecting αβ T cells against cancer cells by transfer of a broadly tumor-reactive γδT-cell receptor. Blood. 2011;118(1):50-9. DOI: 10.1182/blood-2010-12-325993.

[71] Reagan MR, Mishima Y, Glavey SV, Zhang Y, Manier S, Lu ZN, Memarzadeh M, Zhang Y, Sacco A, Aljawai Y, Shi J, Tai YT, Ready JE, Kaplan DL, Roccaro AM, Ghobrial IM. Investigating osteogenic differentiation in multiple myeloma using a novel 3D bone marrow niche model. Blood. 2014;124(22):3250-9. DOI: 10.1182/blood-2014-02-558007.

[72] Fairfield H, Falank C, Farrell M, Vary C, Boucher JM, Driscoll H, Liaw L, Rosen CJ, Reagan MR. Development of a 3D bone marrow adipose tissue model. Bone. 2019;118:77-88. DOI: 10.1016/j.bone.2018.01.023.

[73] Nguyen NT, Shaegh SA, Kashaninejad N, Phan DT. Design, fabrication and characterization of drug delivery systems based on lab-on-a-chip technology. Adv Drug Deliv Rev. 2013;65(11-12):1403-19. DOI: 10.1016/j.addr.2013.05.008.

[74] Torisawa YS, Spina CS, Mammoto T, Mammoto A, Weaver JC, Tat T, Collins JJ, Ingber DE. Bone marrow-on-a-chip replicates hematopoietic niche physiology in vitro. Nat Methods. 2014;11(6):663-9. DOI: 10.1038/nmeth.2938.

[75] Young EW, Pak C, Kahl BS, Yang DT, Callander NS, Miyamoto S, Beebe DJ. Microscale functional cytomics for studying hematologic cancers. Blood. 2012;119(10):e76-85. DOI: 10.1182/blood-2011-10-384347.

[76] Pak C, Callander NS, Young EW, Titz B, Kim K, Saha S, Chng K, Asimakopoulos F, Beebe DJ, Miyamoto S. MicroC(3): an ex vivo microfluidic cis-coculture assay to test chemosensitivity and resistance of patient multiple myeloma cells. Integr Biol (Camb). 2015;7(6):643-54. DOI: 10.1039/c5ib00071h.

[77] Navran S. The application of low shear modeled microgravity to 3-D cell biology and tissue engineering. Biotechnol Annu Rev. 2008;14:275-96. DOI: 10.1016/S1387-2656(08)00011-2.

[78] Grimm D, Wehland M, Pietsch J, Aleshcheva G, Wise P, van Loon J, Ulbrich C, Magnusson NE, Infanger M, Bauer J. Growing tissues in real and simulated microgravity: new methods for tissue engineering. Tissue Eng Part B Rev. 2014;20(6):555-66. DOI: 10.1089/ten.TEB.2013.0704.

[79] Cosmi F, Steimberg N, Dreossi D, Mazzoleni G. Structural analysis of rat bone explants kept in vitro in simulated microgravity conditions. J Mech Behav Biomed Mater. 2009;2(2):164-72. DOI: 10.1016/j.jmbbm.2008.06.004.

[80] Ferrarini M, Steimberg N, Ponzoni M, Belloni D, Berenzi A, Girlanda S, Caligaris-Cappio F, Mazzoleni G, Ferrero E. Ex-vivo

dynamic 3-D culture of human tissues in the RCCS™ bioreactor allows the study of Multiple Myeloma biology and response to therapy. PLoS One. 2013;8(8):e71613. DOI: 10.1371/journal.pone.0071613.

[81] Belloni D, Heltai S, Ponzoni M, Villa A, Vergani B, Pecciarini L, Marcatti M, Girlanda S, Tonon G, Ciceri F, Caligaris-Cappio F, Ferrarini M, Ferrero E. Modeling multiple myeloma-bone marrow interactions and response to drugs in a 3D surrogate microenvironment. Haematologica. 2018;103(4):707-716. DOI: 10.3324/haematol.2017.167486.

[82] Noborio-Hatano K, Kikuchi J, Takatoku M, Shimizu R, Wada T, Ueda M, Nobuyoshi M, Oh I, Sato K, Suzuki T, Ozaki K, Mori M, Nagai T, Muroi K, Kano Y, Furukawa Y, Ozawa K. Bortezomib overcomes cell-adhesion-mediated drug resistance through downregulation of VLA-4 expression in multiple myeloma. Oncogene. 2009;28(2):231-42. DOI: 10.1038/onc.2008.385.

[83] Frenquelli M, Caridi N, Antonini E, Storti F, Viganò V, Gaviraghi M, Occhionorelli M, Bianchessi S, Bongiovanni L, Spinelli A, Marcatti M, Belloni D, Ferrero E, Karki S, Brambilla P, Martinelli-Boneschi F, Colla S, Ponzoni M, DePinho RA, Tonon G. The WNT receptor ROR2 drives the interaction of multiple myeloma cells with the microenvironment through AKT activation. Leukemia. 2020;34(1):257-270. DOI: 10.1038/s41375-019-0486-9

[84] Botrugno OA, Bianchessi S, Zambroni D, Frenquelli M, Belloni D, Bongiovanni L, Girlanda S, Di Terlizzi S, Ferrarini M, Ferrero E, Ponzoni M, Marcatti M, Tonon G. ATR addiction in multiple myeloma: synthetic lethal approaches exploiting established therapies, Haematologica (e-pub ahead of print)

[85] Thompson PA, Burger JA. Bruton's tyrosine kinase inhibitors: first and second generation agents for patients with Chronic Lymphocytic Leukemia (CLL). Expert Opin Investig Drugs. 2018;27(1):31-42. DOI: 10.1080/13543784.2018.1404027.

[86] Barbaglio F, Belloni D, Scarfò L, Sbrana FV, Ponzoni M, Bongiovanni L, Pavesi L, Zambroni D, Stamatopoulos K, Caiolfa VR, Ferrero E, Ghia P, Scielzo C. 3D co-culture model of chronic lymphocytic leukemia bone marrow microenvironment predicts patient-specific response to mobilizing agents. Haematologica. 2020 Jul 30:haematol.2020.248112. DOI: 10.3324/haematol.2020.248112. Epub ahead of print.

[87] Bonomi A, Steimberg N, Benetti A, Berenzi A, Alessandri G, Pascucci L, Boniotti J, Coccè V, Sordi V, Pessina A, Mazzoleni G. Paclitaxel-releasing mesenchymal stromal cells inhibit the growth of multiple myeloma cells in a dynamic 3D culture system. Hematol Oncol. 2017;35(4):693-702. DOI: 10.1002/hon.2306.

[88] Yasui H, Ishida T, Maruyama R, Nojima M, Ikeda H, Suzuki H, Hayashi T, Shinomura Y, Imai K. Model of translational cancer research in multiple myeloma. Cancer Sci. 2012;103(11):1907-12. DOI: 10.1111/j.1349-7006.2012.02384.x.

[89] Brancato V, Oliveira JM, Correlo VM, Reis RL, Kundu SC. Could 3D models of cancer enhance drug screening? Biomaterials. 2020 Feb;232:119744. doi: 10.1016/j.biomaterials.2019.119744. Epub 2019 Dec 26. PMID: 31918229.

[90] Villa A, Belloni D, Vergani B, Cenci S, Cavalli G, Biavasco R, Rodolfo M, Cangi MG, Doglioni C, Dagna L, Ferrero E, Ferrarini M. 3D culture of Erdheim-Chester disease tissues unveils

histiocyte metabolism as a new therapeutic target. Ann Rheum Dis. 2019;78(6):862-864. DOI: 10.1136/annrheumdis-2018-214432.

[91] Calimeri T, Battista E, Conforti F, Neri P, Di Martino MT, Rossi M, Foresta U, Piro E, Ferrara F, Amorosi A, Bahlis N, Anderson KC, Munshi N, Tagliaferri P, Causa F, Tassone P. A unique three-dimensional SCID-polymeric scaffold (SCID-synth-hu) model for in vivo expansion of human primary multiple myeloma cells. Leukemia. 2011:707-11. DOI 10.1038/leu.2010.300.